Eat Meat

And

Stop Jogging

'COMMON' ADVICE ON HOW TO GET FIT IS
KEEPING YOU FAT AND MAKING YOU SICK

Mike Sheridan

Eat Meat And Stop Jogging/Mike Sheridan
ISBN: 978-0993745546
contact@leanlivinginc.com

Contents

This book is dedicated to my parents' generation – the baby boomers. You will continue to struggle if you refuse to abandon the conventional wisdom that's failed you. With an open mind, you can get better!

"A lot of the public is completely unaware that the strength of the message is not matched by the strength of the evidence."

— Barnett Kramer

The Common Trap

The majority of us only ask 'why' when it's abnormal, or challenges our opinion. This opinion, is based on what we've learned in childhood from coaches, teachers, and parents, and further developed by medical professionals, the government, and the media. Forming what we believe is fact, regardless of the credibility of the source and the validity of the information. These so-called 'fundamentals' determine our daily decisions, and help us make choices based on what we think we know is right or wrong and good or bad.

> **Illusion of Truth** – the tendency to believe something is true, the more we hear it.

When it comes to nutrition and exercise, we follow the same advice today as 50 years ago. Despite clear evidence that the original message is seriously flawed, and has contributed to the highest obesity and degenerative disease rates in history. Not only have these false recommendations dominated our day-to-day eating and training habits, but they've determined what we think is necessary to effectively shed the pounds and improve our health. It usually goes something like this:

> *"I just need to eat less and exercise more. It comes down to discipline, you know."*
>
> *"I eat too many fats. I'll cut down on my red meat intake, and start using margarine instead of butter."*
>
> *"I have this friend, and all she did was drink this meal replacement shake for breakfast and she lost 20lbs. I'm going to try that."*
>
> *"I heard that men my age should eat more fiber to lower cholesterol. I'll add an extra serving of whole grains at dinner, and start eating high fiber cereal for breakfast like the Heart Association says I should."*
>
> *"I'm eating too many calories. I'll switch to those 100 calorie snacks between breakfast and dinner, and start incorporating tofu and other plant source proteins instead of meat."*

As you'll learn shortly, there is a reason we believe and follow certain recommendations on nutrition and exercise, like the ones above.

Cognitive fluency – the tendency to believe what's familiar and easy.

Although it's quite obvious that the result of conventional wisdom is making obesity and degenerative disease all too 'common,' many will still have trouble embracing the 'uncommon' advice found in this book. The reality is, common doesn't mean correct, healthy, or sustainable; and obesity, heart disease, Alzheimer's, and cancer don't have to be 'part of the natural aging process.' In the pages that follow, I'll tell you exactly WHY everyone else eats, everyone else says, and everyone else believes certain nutrition and training advice that has unfortunately become common knowledge.

What's driven me to write this book is that over the years I've watched conventional wisdom negatively affect the results of at least 50% of my clients, and ruin the health and body composition of the majority of those around me. I've determined that all I can do to make a difference is communicate what's wrong with the common approach, using over a decade of personal study and experience with clients from all walks of life. I came up with this list of 10 mistakes based on the questions and comments I get most frequently from friends and family, and unfortunately continue to hear from supposed 'experts' online, in magazines and books, and on television. The misunderstanding of topics like calories, saturated fat, cardio, fiber, and cholesterol is negatively affecting daily decision making and leading to an increased likelihood of obesity and disease.

> In the year 2000, 65% of U.S. adults were overweight and 30% obese.
>
> 33% of the U.S. population born after the year 2000 will be diabetic.

Not only is flawed information making and keeping you fat, but it's shortening your life span and increasing your risk of degenerative diseases like cancer, diabetes, Alzheimer's and heart disease.

As you review the mistakes, you'll quickly notice that nearly every piece of misleading information has an ulterior motive. Mainly because the ones with the money run the ads and shout from the rooftops, and this leaves us with tainted day-to-day advice. Despite the current health crisis, government and medical decisions continue to be based on the almighty dollar. My goal is to arm you with the right information so you can recognize and ignore the mass marketing from food manufacturers and corporately funded government projects.

You're here because common advice is not working for you. I know this, because it's not working for anyone. The good news is, once you've read through the 10 mistakes in *Eat Meat And Stop Jogging*, and recognize what's wrong with the current guidelines, I'll show you exactly what's right, while delivering it in a simple and sustainable plan. Experience has taught me that your success with my eating strategy, *Live It NOT Diet!*, will depend on your full understanding of why these bogus recommendations continue and how they're preventing you from optimal health and performance.

It's critical that you continue reading with an open mind as my book opposes many traditional beliefs and several government and medical recommendations. Likely half of you reading this are runners, cyclists, or vegetarians, and you picked up my book because of the title. All I ask is that you take an honest look at the potential future health consequences of your decision to live without animal protein, or rely on endurance exercise to stay fit.

> "There are three things in life that induce powerful visceral responses – religion, politics, and nutrition. Each is based on assumptions, and the adherents of each want to believe in their

hearts that they are right; and of course they refuse to be confused by the facts." Barry Sears, Author of The Zone

After opening your eyes to the mistakes you're making, by laying out the facts, showing you the science, and drawing reasonable conclusions on why certain strategies are flawed, I hope you will continue your journey and start travelling down the correct path with *Live It NOT Diet!*

"I have never seen a person who died of old age. In fact, I do not think that anyone has ever died of old age yet. We invariably die because one vital part has worn out too early in proportion to the rest of the body."

— Dr. Hans Selye (1907-1982)

Restricting Calories To Lose Weight

It is still universally accepted that someone trying to get in shape is seeking 'weight loss.' Despite the fact that scale weight is a poor measure of body composition and a misleading assessment of health. For instance, a woman that weighs 154lbs could be 120lbs of lean mass (bone, tissue, and muscle) and only 34lbs of fat; while another woman could be the same weight (154lbs), but 90lbs of lean mass, and 64lbs of fat.

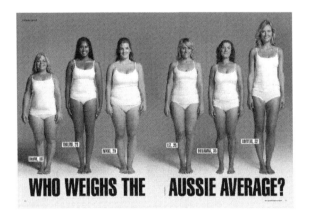

WHO WEIGHS THE AUSSIE AVERAGE?

Weight supplies no information with respect to muscle and fat, and definitely provides no feedback with respect to how we look and feel.

When you speak to most people about their fitness aspirations, it's clear that 'fat loss' is the prevalent goal. Most are looking to lose excess fat, yet they continue to follow strategies that produce drastic amounts of weight loss in a short period of time. Aside from being ineffective and lacking sustainability, this approach is damaging over time. Mainly because weight loss results in muscle loss:

> Research suggests that with a generic weight loss program, muscle loss could be as high as 40% of total weight lost.

As I'll demonstrate in the next section, muscle loss lowers our fat burning rate, increases our fat storage rate, and makes fat loss more difficult over time. Furthermore, it produces a less attractive physique, increases the likelihood of injury and sickness, and accelerates the aging process.

> By seeking weight loss, we look worse, feel worse, lose less fat and make staying fit more difficult in the future than it has to be.

Gaining and maintaining muscle should be prioritized in your quest for a better body and a longer life. Not only because it equates to a higher metabolic (burning) rate, and a more attractive physique, but because muscle loss is associated with aging:

- Slow Phase – 25-50yrs old = 10% loss
- Rapid Phase – 50-80yrs old = 40% loss

By the age of 80, you will have lost nearly 50% of your muscle!

Women seem to battle the muscle maintenance recommendation the most, even though they're the ones most at risk of osteoporosis (a decrease in bone mass and density). Perhaps if they were aware that bone loss is a result of a lack of strength and muscle, they would reevaluate their mindset. Other than an obsession with the scale, this usually stems from the misconception that focusing on activities that build muscle will make women look like a man, or a bodybuilder.

Trust me, female bodybuilders that make me look like Ronald Weesly (the skinny red headed kid from Harry Potter) are not going at it naturally

If you have female friends and acquaintances that lift weights and look bulky, it's because they don't eat right. Compared to a female, males have as much as 8 times the blood concentration of testosterone, and 20 times the daily production. More importantly, if it were easy to naturally bulk up like a bodybuilder, why do most men that lift weights look slim and trim, despite extremely intense lifting schedules and supplementation?

People that work on muscle building and maintenance always look better than those that worry about cutting weight. Not only because a toned muscular build and shape is more aesthetically pleasing, but because muscle increases the rate at which we burn fat.

A Calorie is NOT a Calorie

When weight loss is the goal, caloric restriction is usually the strategy. Largely because this remains the customary advice from fitness and nutrition experts; despite extensive scientific support suggesting otherwise. For instance, here's a recent quote from the President of the International Association for the Study of Obesity:

> "Thinking that a specific diet should eliminate people's weight problems is totally unrealistic, there is no getting around the laws of thermodynamics."

Essentially saying that losing weight is a battle of Calories-In vs. Calories-Out, and has nothing to do with what 'type' of food we eat. As well as implying that individuals are obese because they eat too much and don't exercise enough. As my personal results demonstrate and the following research proves, this guidance is severely flawed.

In 1890, a chemist named Wilbur Atwater discovered that the amount of energy in food could be determined by burning food to ash (in a device called the calorimeter) and measuring the heat produced. According to Atwater:

> One calorie equals the amount of heat required to raise the temperature of one gram of water by one degree.

Surprisingly, this is still the measurement used today to determine the calorie content in different foods. The question is, does it seem reasonable to say that our body operates just like Wilbur's oven?

Does it make sense to think that nothing else determines if we store or lose fat?

If that were the case, one would expect 3 unique diets with the same total calories to produce identical results in weight-loss, right?

Fortunately, researchers in 1957 did just that. They put participants on 1 of 3 1000-calorie diets, varying the percentages of each macronutrient with either 90% fat, 90% carbs, or 90% protein.

The 90% protein and 90% fat groups lost between 0.6 and 0.9 lbs per day, while the 90% carb group actually gained!

Calorie Restriction = Muscle Mass Loss

What the misguided calorie restriction experts believe and promote is that you lose weight by either:
- Lowering your caloric intake = eat less
- Increasing your energy expenditure = exercise more

Will this make you lose weight? Yes.
Will you lose weight fast? Yes.

Is all of this weight fat? No.
Is it healthy? No.
Is it sustainable? No.

Weight loss is unfavorable if a good portion of it is muscle. Generally, this is the case with calorie restriction strategies as there's no stipulation other than 'eat less.' To illustrate this point, lets look at interesting research from 2010 that compared 3 diets with varying amounts of protein:

- Low Protein – 5% protein, 52% fat, 42% carbs
- Normal Protein – 15% protein, 44% fat, and 42% carbs
- High Protein – 25% protein, 33% fat, 41% carbs

The great thing about this study is that its initial premise was to show that eating too many calories causes fat gain regardless of food choice; which it appeared to accomplish, as all participants gained 8lbs of fat. However, when we take a more thorough look at the data it's clear that the composition of that weight gain is quite different:

> The low protein group gained least total body weight, but along with 8lbs of fat, they lost 1.5lbs in muscle mass.
>
> The normal and high protein groups gained muscle mass, approximately 6lbs and 7.5lbs respectively.

Although the weight gain was higher in the normal and high protein groups, nearly half of that was useful, healthy, and metabolically active muscle mass. The composition of the input was different, and so was the composition of the output. When looking at strictly body composition, the high protein group produced the most impressive outcome. They stored only 50% of the excess calories as fat, and stored the other 50% as lean muscle mass.

The low-protein group stored >90% as fat and lost muscle!

Calorie Restriction = Slower Metabolism (RMR)

The research above not only shows us that a lack of protein causes muscle mass loss, but it supplies another very important piece of information:

> The low-protein group had a 2% decrease in Resting Metabolic Rate (RMR), while the normal & high-protein groups had an 11% Increase in RMR.

Essentially, this means that:

> *When sedentary (inactive) the low-protein group will burn less calories per day because of a slower Resting Metabolic Rate.*

Nearly 75% of our total energy expenditure is determined by our Resting Metabolic Rate (RMR); meaning a low rate can be extremely detrimental. On a calorie restriction plan, the RMR drops because of a lack of energy in, and muscle loss. The reason there's muscle loss is because the foods that facilitate muscle maintenance are usually restricted to meet the caloric constraints. In other words, when someone operates in a caloric deficit they continue to decrease the rate at which they burn calories, and lose useful muscle that would otherwise have burned additional calories.

Prolonged caloric reduction (3100kcal to 1950kcal) decreases metabolic rate by 20% per kg of bodyweight

24 weeks of severe caloric restriction decreases metabolic rate by 40%

25

Unfortunately, those following these strategies are left eating less but gaining more, because of their slowed metabolism. What's more, is that once their metabolic rate drops, it can take a significant amount of time to bring back to its pre-diet level.

"But it was only a 6 week bikini season shred-up. I'll return to normal and I'll do it again after Christmas? My body's rate will go back up and start living normal again, right?"

During the restoration period following a calorie-restricted diet the threshold to gain is much lower. The reduced burning rate means less intake will be required to create a surplus. A decreased metabolic rate also lowers the absorption of muscle building foods, like protein. Implying that if a standard diet is reestablished, the synthesis of these essential foods is diminished.

Considering that our body reduces its metabolic rate as we age, by approximately 2.3% per decade after the age of 20, the outcome from a lifetime of dieting is extremely unfortunate.

Calorie Restriction = Hormone Disruption

The worst outcome from calorie restriction is that it raises the hormones responsible for hunger and fat storage, and lowers or inhibits the hormones that suppress hunger and promote fat burning.

Calorie restriction increases fat storage hormones, and decreases fat burning hormones.

Equally disturbing, is that similar to our metabolic rate, it appears that this disruption in hormones lasts for a substantial time period after the restriction phase. For example, a 2011 study in the New England Journal of Medicine determined that after a 10-week period of restricting calories, not only did hunger and fat storage hormones elevate, but leptin (the hormone that prevents fat storage) remained low for a FULL YEAR!

Low leptin not only promotes fat storage, but research has suggested that:

A 20% decrease in leptin produces a 24% increase in hunger!

Ghrelin is the hunger hormone, and when leptin is down ghrelin is up. Upon completion of a calorie restriction diet, you are burning less (low metabolism), storing more (low leptin), and hungrier (high ghrelin). Other than leptin, you're looking at a reduction in thyroid hormone (t3) and the sympathetic nervous system, which are driving forces in lowering your overall metabolic rate. Many think that our thyroid hormone is the major determinant of metabolism, until they learn that leptin controls the thyroid.

When a calorie-restricted diet is your strategy to lose, it becomes harder and harder to keep the fat off. Although you may lose 'weight' in the short-term, the negative hormonal consequences produce a lifelong struggle.

Calorie Restriction = Decreased Satiation

One of the reasons many fail on diets and calorie restriction plans is because they're constantly hungry. Although ghrelin (the hunger hormone) plays a major part, it's largely because our body is seeking nutritionally dense food for proper functioning. A meal high in animal protein not only supplies cells with what they require, but it increases fullness and satisfaction until lunch, and decreases the motivation for food throughout the day. On a calorie restriction plan, a meal containing animal protein would be frowned upon, because it's high in calories. After a meal like this, individuals on a diet would likely have to restrict their intake for the rest of the day in order to avoid going over in 'points.' Those following such an approach have been severely misguided, as we require the essential fats, nutrients, and amino acids in these food sources for survival. Not only are we fighting one of our basic primal desires to consume these high-calorie foods, and missing out on higher levels of satiation (fullness), but we're putting our health and longevity at risk.

Despite efforts to lower calories and restrict higher calorie fats and proteins in North America, obesity has nearly tripled. It appears we've been listening to the message, but we're clearly not getting the result. For instance, take a look at the change in % of food 'type' from 1965 to 1991 in teenagers in the U.S. (11-18 years):

	1965	1977	1989-1991
Total Energy (mJ)	9.92	8.78	8.77
% from fat	38.7	37.0	34.3
% from sat fat	15.0	14.1	12.9
% from carb	46.3	47.1	51.4
% from protein	16.1	16.7	15.4

Total calories, fat and protein have all decreased, yet obesity has steadily increased over the same time period. This is because it's not the number of calories in a meal, it's the quality of those calories. There are specific foods that build muscle, burn fat, and support our health and longevity, but conventional wisdom tells us to exclude these foods if we're attempting to get in shape. Sadly, the long-term affect from this approach leads to a consistent struggle to get fit and remain disease-free.

Calorie Restriction = Unhealthy

Failing to provide our body with adequate nutrients in an effort to eat less calories causes deficiency and degeneration. For instance, by limiting fats because they are the highest calorically (9kcal vs. 4kcal in carbohydrates and protein) we inhibit the absorption of essential fat-soluble nutrients (A, D, E, and K) and the synthesis of key steroid hormones (testosterone, estrogen, androgen). Our body needs these nutrients to manufacture, repair, and refurbish our bone, tissue, and cartilage, and the cells of the heart, brain, and liver. Failing to provide this ongoing nutritional support over time leads to deterioration and cell death, and damage associated with aging and disease.

When food is scarce, mammals utilize the limited supply of energy they have to survive; and this forces other systems to go dormant. Research has suggested that when food and nutrient supply (or caloric intake) is inadequate to meet metabolic demands, the reproductive system can suffer - leading to puberty and development delays, ovulation suppression, testosterone reduction, and an increased risk of infertility. It also harms physical strength and performance, especially when the reduction in calories is excessive.

Calorie Restriction Weight Loss = NOT Sustainable

If you're anything like the majority, you are making a concentrated effort to get and stay fit. Unfortunately, the same misconceptions that landed you in the overweight or obese category are preventing you from getting out. You either continue to lose weight and gain it back, or have yo-yo'd so many times you're now incapable of losing any to begin with. As I've illustrated, this is because a chronic caloric deficit results in muscle loss, an increase in fat storage hormones, and a reduced metabolic rate.

> You may be fooling the scale (and yourself) in the short-term, but you will not sustain the weight loss, and in the long-run you're only harming your health.

Although many can and will enjoy a significant amount of 'weight' loss on a calorie restriction diet, they eventually regain. What's worse, is that they tend to gain more than when they started, because their 'gain fat' threshold is reduced. Generally, they're heavier than their pre-diet weight; and sadly, a greater proportion of it is fat. This is not only frustrating, as they've put in significant effort, but it's depressing, as the advice from so-called experts suggests they are to blame.

> The day you stop reducing calories to lose, is the day you start losing without reducing calories.

There's an easier way to get and stay fit, and it doesn't require eating like a bird and exercising like a maniac. The reason extreme dieters continue to struggle, is because they continue to go on extreme diets. They lose a ton of weight, regain a ton of weight, and have to work twice as hard to lose 'any' weight in the future. As I will continue to show you, it's not the number of calories in a meal, it's the quality and composition of those calories.

"Vegan and vegetarian children often fail to grow as well as their omnivorous cohorts despite apparently adequate intakes of amino acids and nitrogen."

— Dr. Loren Cordain

Limiting or Avoiding Animal Protein

When you put nutrient dense food in your body, you get superior performance in return. Similar to premium fuel in an engine, this also prevents the need for future repairs. Unfortunately, many are missing out on essential nutrients because the foods highest in calories are also the foods that provide the most benefit. The perfect example is animal protein, which is both high in calories and high in nutrients. Sadly, the last 40 years have created other reasons to avoid meat that extend far beyond calories. Although the rationale is equally misunderstood, the impact on our health and body composition is far more damaging.

To best illustrate the consequences of restricting or avoiding a premium fuel like animal protein, we'll take a look at vegetarians. A reliance on plant-based protein alternatives leaves non-meat eaters malnourished, and deficient in essential fatty acids (omega-3), vitamins (D, B12, E, A) and several essential amino acids.

> When foods are 'essential' it means they can only be acquired in the diet; meaning if you're not eating them, you're not getting them!

A lack of adequate nutrition from animal source foods leads to less muscle mass and an increased risk of degenerative disease. As mentioned in Mistake #1, our muscle mass determines our metabolic rate, but it also influences our long-term health. Limiting animal protein may only lead to minor deficiencies (like anemia) in the short-term, but this can quickly develop into osteoporosis, and Alzheimer's as we age.

Humans Need Animal Protein

Could you kill an animal with a knife, rock, or even your bare hands?

The truth is, not a lot of us could. Not only because we've never had to but because we know it would be challenging, physically and psychologically.

So, if we are perfectly capable of surviving on roots, shoots, nuts and berries, what drove the human beings before us to track and kill an animal?

What gave them the desire to make a spear and risk their life battling a saber-toothed tiger or wooly mammoth?

I'd say the innate need for the essential nutrients, amino acids, and fats from animal flesh. They recognized that this food source was a necessity in providing their family with the essentials of life.

> Failure to consume meat leads to nutritional deficiencies just like it did 1.5 million years ago in our hominoid ancestors.

My research and experience has taught me that the decision to eliminate or replace animal protein is the biggest mistake one can make in an effort to improve their physique and long-term health. Yes, there are 'other protein options,' but they are incomplete, and lack the essential vitamins, fatty-acids, minerals, and amino acids required to remain strong, energized, and disease-free.

> There are many that will survive without animal protein, but they will not thrive.

Sadly, those surviving without animal protein may not recognize the negative effects until it's already too late.

Plant Protein Does NOT = Animal Protein

There's an endless supply of books from former vegans sharing their personal story of a slow decline in health, and their plea to confused vegetarians to change their ways. Interestingly, a lot of the nutrition experts of today are former vegetarians, like Chris Masterjohn and Robb Wolf, who have the desire to share their story to make sure others don't make the same mistakes. It may be difficult to open your mind to a carnivore like me, so if you're looking for more in depth information take a look at two of my favorite reads:

'The Vegetarian Myth' and 'The Whole Soy Story.'

One of the biggest and most common threats from a reliance on plant source proteins is the risk of B12 deficiency; as it can only properly be obtained from animal source foods. Unfortunately, B12 is especially finicky when it comes to absorption, as proper stomach acid (hydrochloric acid and the intrinsic factor) is required for sufficient breakdown and uptake. In other words, it's not just a lack of B12 containing meat, but rather the continuous decline in stomach acid because of inactivity. When animal protein is finally consumed, the underactive stomach secretes less acid and can't effectively break down the food to access the nutrients. Leaving non-meat-eaters with less absorption of essential nutrients from animal source foods. Sadly, the digestive discomfort experienced when low-mat eaters finally decide to eat meat gives many the false reassurance that they shouldn't be eating it. B12 deficiency is an extremely common diagnosis for young females (along with iron deficiency), as most of them don't eat nearly enough animal protein. Other than low energy, many won't recognize the symptoms or negative impact of deficiency until it's too late.

A lack of B12 is associated with a shrinking brain, and accelerated aging rate.

Anemia, or low-iron, is said to be the most common nutritional deficiency in North America. I believe this is largely influenced by a universal fear of meat. Heme (or ferrous) is the best iron source available to us as human beings and it's the most absorbable. Unfortunately, for those limiting or replacing animal protein, heme iron is only obtainable from meat, and is more absorbable when meat is present in the meal. This topic is especially important for menstruating females, as they're experiencing significant monthly blood loss and tend to eat less red meat in general.

Omega-3 essential fatty acids (DHA & EPA) are the third source of deficient nutrition in a diet lacking animal protein. Plant, or non-meat protein options only contain ALA, which has to be successfully converted to DHA to supply any benefit. Unfortunately:

> Attempting to raise blood DHA status with strictly an ALA source is nearly impossible!

Similar to B12, a lack of DHA is associated with declining cognitive and behavioral performance. As you'll learn in Mistake #3 and #5, the flawed advice for North Americans to restrict saturated fat in favor of plant oils (omega-6s), inhibits ALA conversion even further. For vegans this is of extreme concern, as most consume no saturated fat and rely heavily on plant protein sources that are high in omega-6 polyunsaturated fats.

> The non-meat omega-3, ALA, has been shown to raise prostate cancer, while the animal source variety (DHA & EPA) lowers it!

Believing that tofu, quinoa, soy, pinto beans, and brown rice can give you everything that animal protein provides, is an extremely flawed mindset. The Rancho Bernardo Study from 2002 looked at the consumption of different types of protein in 970 men and women between 55 and 92 years of age. Researchers determined that animal protein sources were positively correlated with bone mineral density, while vegetable sources were negatively correlated. Another study compared the health of 2 prehistoric populations living in the same area but with very unique diets. The Hardin Villagers lived mainly on corn, beans, and squash, and the hunter-gatherers (the Indian Knoll) mostly meat, fish, and wild fruit. After researchers analyzed the health of both populations, this is what they found:

- Longer lifespan and lower infant mortality (from malnutrition) for the hunter-gatherers
- Common iron, calcium, and protein deficiencies in the villagers – none in the hunter-gatherers
- No bone malformations or cavities in the hunter-gatherers, versus an average of 7 for the farmers

---

Soy = Toxic

Soy is often regarded as the 'vegetarian answer' to a diet lacking muscle-building protein.   Apparently tofu and other soy alternatives provide just as much benefit as animal protein.

Fact 1: A safe amount of soy is only 36g per day, and a single block of tofu contains 250g.

We're also told that Orientals eat a lot of soy, and that's why they're healthier than North Americans.

Fact 2: The Japanese and Chinese treat soy as a condiment, and usually consume in it's safest form – fermented.

In the 1930's in China, total soy consumption was 1.5% of calories, while pork was 65%!

A 1998 study in Taka Yama City, Japan, reviewed soy consumption from 1242 men and 3596 women, and determined that the daily intake averaged 3-13g/day for men, and 3-11g/day for women.

The reason you think eating soy like the Japanese will lower your risk of heart disease is because that's what you've been told by companies that sell soy. What you'll learn shortly is that saturated fat and red meat are not to blame for heart disease, and promoting soy as a health food because it lowers cholesterol is a misguided message to begin with.

Relying on a toxic substance as your main or dominant protein source can have a highly damaging impact on your health. Everyone loves stats, so here are 4 of my favorites:

> *Men who consumed the equivalent of one cup of soy milk per day had a 50% lower sperm count than men who had none.*

> *In 1992, the Swiss Health Service estimated that two cups of soy milk per day provides the estrogenic equivalent of one birth control pill.*

> *Infants exclusively fed soy formula receive the estrogenic equivalent (based on body weight) of at least 5 birth control pills PER DAY!*

> *A Study on the brains of 4000 Hawaiian Men determined that men who ate the most tofu had smaller brains and double the risk of developing Alzheimer's.*

These are the statistics for a food regarded as 'healthy' and superior to animal products for disease prevention.

Soy = Disrupted Hormones

As perhaps you recognized while reading the 4 statistics in the last section, soy has a negative hormonal impact on the body. Phytoestrogens are plants hormones found in soy that mimic the natural human/animal hormone 'estrogen,' and bind to estrogen receptor sites. Although it's a typical reaction to think of estrogen as a female hormone, this discussion is applicable to both sexes. These estrogen mimickers (or xenoestrogens) - also found in cosmetics, pesticides, plastics, insecticides, and environmental pollutant - are said to be a contributing factor in the development of estrogen-dominant cancers (breast and prostate). In a nutshell, this toxic substance, that originally evolved in plants as a defense mechanism to inhibit reproductive health, is able to live in your body and cause huge problems.

Our largest intake of phytoestrogens comes from soybean oil and other common additives (sunflower, cottonseed, safflower), which as you'll discover in Mistake #5, are called polyunsaturated fatty-acids (PUFAs). The use of these oils has skyrocketed, as we've been conned into choosing low-fat foods. Despite being toxic to humans and livestock, the most common use of soybeans in North America is as a vegetable oil additive in packaged foods and animal feed.

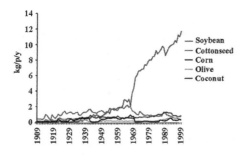

"The estimated per capita consumption of soybean oil increased more than 1000-fold from 1909 to 1999."

One can see the immediate negative impact this 'fake estrogen' can have on men, as it competes with testosterone for receptor sites and can display itself in the form of 'man-boobs,' and other non-manly characteristics. An estrogen overload in women is less obvious, although equally as damaging. Over time, excess estrogen can lead to infertility, breast and prostate cancer, and endocrine disruption.

Isoflavones are also found in soy, and like phytoestrogens they interrupt regular hormone functioning. The production of thyroid hormone, which usually regulates how the body uses energy and grows, is disrupted by isoflavones. As Dr. Kaayla Daniels explains in The Whole Soy Story, the isoflavones produce a hyperactive thyroid at first, which means energy levels and metabolic rate elevate. Although, over time the isoflavones facilitate a hypoactive thyroid, which leads to fat storage, hair loss, and poor energy. This could explain why some mention feeling fantastic when replacing other proteins with soy protein, or adding soy to their diet; when clearly, the experience is short-lived.

> "A Japanese study at the Ishizuki Clinic found that just 35mg of isoflavones per day caused thyroid suppression in healthy individuals in just three months....a glass of soy milk contains about 45mg." – Dr. Kaayla Daniels, *The Whole Soy Story*

The U.S. economy and many BIG businesses, like Monsanto, have a lot invested in the success of soy.

> In the year 2000, the U.S. produced 75 million tons of soybeans, and exported nearly 30% of that.

Similar to the promotion of whole grains as a 'requirement' in a healthy diet (discussed in Mistake #7), we're being misled in an effort to protect economic and corporate interests. For example, research posted in the New England Journal of Medicine in 1995 concluded that the consumption of soy protein lowers cholesterol. The study was financed by a corporation (DuPont Protein Technologies) that produces and markets soy through a sister organization (The Solae Company).

Although there have been attempts to instill the benefits of soy in our minds from corporations, the media, and even the government, it's clear that the evidence supporting the negative impact is far superior.

Legumes = Decreased Absorption & Intestinal Health

Soy is not the only legume that can be harmful to our health when over-consumed. Like grains, nuts, and seeds, legumes come equipped with plant defenses that are designed to prevent consumption. Plants don't have a distinct security system like humans and animals that can immediately resist or inflict harm on initial contact. However, they are quite capable of inflicting considerable damage over time. This slow, and many times unnoticeable, defense system becomes increasingly prevalent when these toxin-packed plants are consumed frequently and in large quantities.

The first problem with legumes is that they contain phytic acid (or phytates), which have been shown to reduce the absorption of magnesium, calcium, iron, zinc, and B12. A vegetarian will tell you that phytates can be avoided with proper preparation procedures (sprouting, soaking, draining, and boiling), but research tells us that only 50% are removed with an 18hr soak. Given the North American norm of prioritizing speed and convenience over quality, it's also highly unlikely that the majority would practice such a tedious process.

> We eat to nourish our bodies with the vitamins, minerals, essential fats and proteins we require to live, so absorption is pivotal.

Ironically, the minerals we fail to absorb in plant-based alternatives are the same ones excluded in a diet devoid of animal protein. In other words, vegetarians are going to extremes to make a food edible that would otherwise not be, when perfectly safe and more nutritious foods (meat) are available.

Legumes are also high in lectins, which can cause intestinal damage, and increase ones risk of an autoimmune disease, like IBS, Crohn's, and Colitis.

> "...lectins can interact with a variety of other cells in the body and are recognized as the major anti-nutrient of food."

Lectins can also bind to insulin receptors; which increases our risk of leptin resistance. As we've discussed, adequate leptin levels are critical in determining our metabolic rate, and suppressing fat storage and hunger hormones. If our cells become resistant to leptin we become more prone to over-eating and under-burning.

Don't get me wrong, other foods have natural defenses, and many foods other than beans are high in lectins. However, problems arise with the over-consumption and over-reliance on these foods as a protein staple. A few soaked beans once in a while isn't going to kill you, but 1 or 2 meals with beans every day and you run the risk of digestion and absorption issues.

Legumes = High in Carbohydrates

The other reason legumes are an inferior protein source is because they are very high in carbohydrates. The first number in the chart below is the glycemic load (blood sugar response), and the second number is the total carbohydrates in 1 cup of some of the most commonly consumed beans:

Pink	68:135	Adzuki	62:124
Mung	59:130	Black	57:121
White	56:122	Pinto	55:121
Chickpeas	52:121	Small White	47:134
Great Northern	46:114	Navy	44:127
French	42:118	Yellow	40:119
Cranberry	40:117	Kidney	37:110
Fava	28:87	Baked Beans	21:55
Soy	19:56	Lima	13:31

As you'll discover shortly (Mistake #6), excess daily carbohydrates are the driving force in body fat gain. When looking at legumes, even the varieties on the lower end (ex: Fava Beans) still contain far too many carbohydrates for 1 serving. are far too high for 1 serving at 1 meal. Although legumes appear to be a viable source

46

of protein for non-meat eaters, an over-reliance on this food (as your primary protein source at most meals) negatively affects your body composition.

Not ALL Meat is Created Equal

Somehow, as I sit here in 2013 I am handed a new diet book from my brother where the author outlines the importance of avoiding animal foods to improve overall health and lose weight. Yet when I read his support for why limiting animal products is 'fundamental,' his points are far from relevant to his recommendations. As per usual, his suggestions carry no reliable scientific support, and he continuously refers to animal protein as 'factory farmed' meat, and classifies meat-eating as pizzas and cheeseburgers.

> *Not all meat is industrially produced, grain-fed, and pumped with antibiotics, just like not all vegetables are Genetically Modified (GMO).*

Grass-fed beef, free-run poultry, and wild fish are easily attainable with a little effort and a minor budget adjustment. In fact, selecting higher quality meat is usually more satiating (filling); which translates to eating less and potentially lowering grocery costs.

> Quality animal protein can be obtained from local farmers with respectable production and treatment processes.

There's also a tendency to group red meat and processed meat together, even though unprocessed red meat continues to show no association with an increase in disease. For example, a 2009 study concluded that:

> "A high consumption of red meat was related to higher all-cause mortality, and the association was stronger for processed meat. **After correction for measurement error**, higher all-cause mortality remained significant only for processed meat."

Processed meat is clearly the issue, just like GMOs and pesticides are in fruits and vegetables. When analyzing foods, it's unfair to look at the very best variety of one you're in favor of, and compare it to the worst variety of the one you're against. That's like saying a hockey team is better because their 1st line center is better than the other team's 3rd line center. If that's the case, the plant-based proteins we should consider when comparing them to animal protein, should be the genetically modified varieties.

> The only time reliable correlations between meat and cancer have been drawn are when processed (sausage, bacon, or cold cuts) or improperly prepared (burnt or charred) meats are used.

We all want to avoid factory-farming, processing, GMOs, pesticides, antibiotics and any other ingredients that harm our health. When comparing dietary choices it's essential to look at the best or equivalent options of each.

Not ALL Meat-Eaters are Created Equal

Vegetarians often refer to The Seventh Day Adventists (a vegetarian Christian group) as an example of low cancer and mortality rates from the avoidance of meat. The problem is, it's unfair to compare this group to a meat-eater in regular society, because The Seventh Day Adventists are a secluded group that doesn't smoke or drink, and likely doesn't engage in other life shortening lifestyle choices. A meat-eating equivalent would be the Mormons, who follow equivalent principles and similar daily practices. When comparing the Mormons risk of cancer and mortality to the U.S. average, the results are equally (if not more) impressive:

- 22% Lower Cancer Risk
- 34% Lower Mortality from Colon Cancer

Furthermore, despite the lower risk of colon cancer for the Seventh Day Adventists, they seem to experience higher rates of other cancers - Hodgkin's disease, malignant melanoma, brain, skin, uterine, prostate, endometrial, cervical, and ovarian.

Over-reliance on plant-based proteins?

Lack of animal protein?

Monocrops = Murder

We are repeatedly told that "grains can feed the world." Although, what many fail to recognize (without revisiting the dietary consequences of a reliance on plant based proteins) is that wheat, corn & soy are Monocrops.

A monocrop is planted, grows, is consumed, and strips the earth of its ability to reproduce. Monocrops increase the rate of soil erosion from ploughing, and decrease the water and nutrient content of the soil.

"A nation that destroys its soil destroys itself." Franklin D. Roosevelt

Once the soil is destroyed in one area, the crop field must occupy a new location (with fertile soil), and significant time and resources are needed to restore the previous site. When you consider the amount of irrigation needed to water these crops, and the land that it occupies, the monocrop footprint is significant. This drives animals out of their homes, and uses up the resources they need to survive.

It's suggested that 90% of the Northern US Prairies have been taken over by monocrops.

We are damaging our land and using up our resources to grow a food that may fill us up, but will not provide proper nourishment. Conversely, 1 cow can nourish 1 human for an entire year, and the cow's relationship with the earth is a renewable one:

Soil – Grass – Cows – Humans – Soil (Repeat)

A cows stomach allows it to consume grass and digest cellulose. We, as humans, cannot digest grass and therefore look to the cow to consume grass and convert it into digestible fat and protein (it's body). The cow is not only providing humans with essential protein and fat, but they're ensuring the health of the grass & soil by:

Grazing - *keeps the grass short and allows it to re-grow properly.*

Fertilizing – *bacteria in the stomach of the cow feed on the grass and the cow consumes the bacteria for growth. When the*

cow digests and eliminates waste, it provides manure to the soil,
which feeds the grass, and fertilizes it with nutrients to grow.

Crops, on the other hand, are occupying and destroying the land, sucking water reserves dry and not promoting regrowth.

The environmental reasoning for not eating meat is severely flawed, and the moral reasoning may be even worse.

Animal Protein = Better Health & Longevity

We need meat to thrive, and as I'll continue to show you, it's an essential requirement for obtaining a lean, muscular physique. Science continues to prove that animal products increase longevity, while the vegetarian diet is correlated with an early grave. A perfect example is the Hindus in Southern India, who have the lowest life expectancy in the world because of a lack of meat in their diet.

The reality is, vegetarians have equal rates of atherosclerosis, and higher mortality rates.

On average, meat-eating women live 32% longer!

Yet, many continue to avoid meat because of unnecessary fears surrounding saturated fat and cholesterol. This misconception runs so deep that I've dedicated the next 2 chapters to clearing it up. I hope you will join me!

"All truth passes through three stages. First, it is ridiculed. Second, it is violently opposed. Third, it is accepted as self-evident."

— Arthur Schopenhauer

Blaming Saturated Fat For Heart Disease

Our hunter-gatherer ancestors, from hundreds of thousands of years ago, thrived averaging 50% of their total calories from animal foods.

> "The prehistoric humans of North America frequented animals such as camel, bison, mammoth, mountain sheep, bear, wild pig, beaver, elk, mule deer, sloth, and antelope, what we'd refer to as 'very fatty meats' today."

When you analyze the tissue of these foods, you'll notice a very high percentage of saturated fats, and an extremely low level of polyunsaturated fats. It's important to note that polyunsaturated fats are what we've been told to increase over the last 50 years to replace saturated fats. The 'experts' have instructed us to restrict or eliminate saturated fats to prevent obesity and disease. Even though the diseases plaguing North Americans over the past 10,000 years were virtually non-existent in fatty-meat eating hunter-gatherers.

Dr. Loren Cordain, a top global researchers in the area of evolutionary medicine, suggests that there was no cancer, diabetes, heart disease, and even near-sightedness and acne in these men and women.

As for obesity, here's the standard physique of those eating 50% of their total calories from animal foods high in saturated fat:

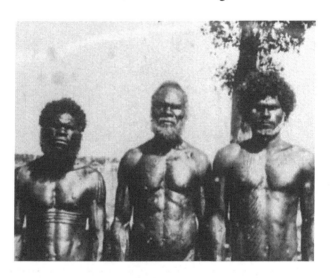

Hunter-gatherers were also taller than most Modern Americans, and without the bone malformations and cavities associated with poor nutrition.

"But didn't Neanderthals and Hunter-Gatherers have a short average life expectancy?"

Yes, but childhood death was more common which skewed the average, and those of the Paleolithic Era had to deal with an inferior shelter, a long-list of hungry predators, and weren't blessed with the convenience of a hospital down the street. Despite having no heath care, one could argue that the infant mortality rate was surprisingly low, and the life expectancy relatively high (10% of them lived into their 60's).

Even if we are living longer now, it's clear that less and less of those years are 'disease-free!'

What we seem to forget is that the last 10,000 years makes up an extremely small amount of time in human history. Robb Wolf puts it perfectly when he relates our human history to a football field, saying that:

> "...if we started walking from one end-zone toward the other, we could walk 99.5 yards, and this would represent all of human history except the last 5000 years or so."

Genetically, there's very little that separates us from our 'healthy' hunter-gatherer ancestors; with some evidence suggesting less than 0.02%. What's changed is our diet. We've gone from humans that favor fat, to humans that fear it.

Saturated Fat Research = Flawed

The recommendation to lower saturated fat was born in the 1950's, when Dr. Ancel Keys presented results from research comparing dietary fat and heart disease in 7 countries. His findings indicated that Americans were eating the most fat and had the highest rate of death from heart disease, while the Japanese were eating the least and had the lowest rate of death.

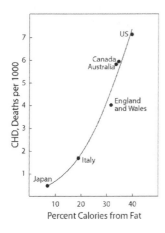

I suppose Ancel was trying to make a name for himself as he conveniently failed to mention that his research was actually performed on 22 countries! When all 22 countries were included, Dr. Key's results showed no significance.

Finland and Mexico ate similar amounts of fat, yet the death rate from heart disease was 24 TIMES HIGHER in Finland!

Unfortunately, once this research was accepted as proof, future experiments continued to cite Key's research and create somewhat of a snowball effect. The originally tainted science was quickly perceived as 'fact,' and the government and health associations started making claims like this:

"High-fat foods are causing coronary heart disease and other deadly problems in Americans, and these high-fat foods are just as dangerous to the public as cigarettes. The depth of the SCIENCE BASE underlying its findings is even more impressive than that of tobacco and health in 1964."

Saturated Fat Does NOT Cause Heart Disease

Similar country comparison research has been done since Keys falsified study. For instance, in 1998 in the journal Nutrition, researchers looked at the average intake of saturated fat in 41 European countries and compared it to the risk of death from heart disease.

The countries with the HIGHEST saturated fat intake had some of the LOWEST death rates from cardiovascular disease; while the lowest intakes (like Georgia and Azerbaijan) had some of the highest rates.

Here's the map of cardiovascular deaths (highest = dark):

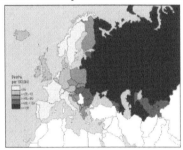

Compared to the map of fat intake (highest = dark):

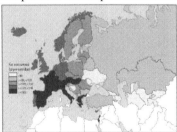

Although it's been proven time-and-time again, but somehow never properly acknowledged, there is no connection between saturated fat and heart disease:

> Switzerland, Belgium, and France eat the most saturated fat (>15% of total calories), and have the lowest heart disease.
>
> Japan and Israel nearly doubled their intake of animal fat after WWII, yet heart disease continues to fall.
>
> France and Finland consume similar amounts of fat, but one has 3 times the heart disease.
>
> Since replacing coconut oil and clarified butter (saturated fats) with vegetable oils, India has gone from the country with the lowest heart disease to the one with the highest.

I know it's still hard to swallow. It seems so simple to believe that fatty meat and butter are to blame; as we can all picture a big slab of butter-coated red meat clogging up our arteries. However, research continues to show that saturated fat is not to blame:

> In 2009, there was a review of 21 studies analyzing the saturated fat intake in a total of 350,000 people; all found NO ASSOCIATION with heart disease!

Even though the evidence is readily available, many still believe we need to lower our fat intake. Mainly because dieticians, governments, and doctors are continue to make claims like this:

> "Saturated fats and dietary cholesterol have no known beneficial role in preventing chronic disease and are not required at any level in the diet." Food and Drug Administration, 2002

Clearly we haven't benefited from this advice. Since the low-fat recommendation were introduced, obesity rates have doubled and heart disease remains the number 1 cause of death in the U.S. We've lowered fat intake nationally, yet we're fatter than ever, and heart disease, diabetes, depression, and cancer rates have skyrocketed.

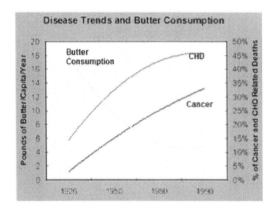

In the year 1900 we averaged 18lbs of butter per person per year, and in 1995 we had less than 5lbs.

Unfortunately, Ancel Keys ridiculous research isn't the only thing feeding our fear of saturated animal fats. The next section covers what could be the biggest façade of them all. Sadly, it's also the most heavily funded, and continues to be spread by a group of highly-trusted foot soldiers.

"Many of today's physicians, originally trained decades ago, don't have a firm grasp of nutrition and its effects on your health...My hope is that our next generation of doctors will be better equipped to swing the pendulum to the side of prevention rather than focus so much on treatment."

— Dr. David Perlmutter

Thinking Cholesterol Causes Heart Disease

The misleading advice on cholesterol stems from similar beginnings to the falsified research on fat. In 1913, a Russian Pathologist named Nikolai Anitschkow was the first to make a clear connection between cholesterol and atherosclerosis. His experiments discovered legions in the arteries of cholesterol-fed rabbits, similar to what is seen in the early stages of atherosclerosis in humans. With the added support from Ancel Key's flawed fat research 40 years later, the medical community was convinced they knew the cause of heart disease:

Saturated Fat = High Cholesterol = Heart Disease

It all made sense, saturated fat raises total cholesterol and this rise in cholesterol is what causes heart disease. Before you could blink, 98% of doctors were on-board in 1978, with what was dubbed 'the lipid hypothesis.'

In 1984, the National Institute of Health gathered 14 experts who voted unanimously that lowering cholesterol reduces coronary heart disease and risk of heart attack.

The lipid hypothesis quickly became fact; and unfortunately the majority of the population has been brainwashed into still believing it today.

High Cholesterol Does NOT = Heart Disease

Despite the support from the medical community, there is significant evidence providing proof that high cholesterol levels do not cause heart disease. As many well-respected doctors and scientists have pointed out, the original data supporting the lipid hypothesis, and countless experiments since are based on "inaccuracies, misinterpretations, exaggerations and misleading quotations in this research area." Furthermore, any scientific support proving a lack of association between mortality and heart disease have been conveniently excluded, and research suggesting a correlation between cholesterol and heart disease are heavily promoted. I suppose when you consider the billions of dollars in profits from the sale of cholesterol lowering statin drugs, this shouldn't come as a surprise.

A study from 2005 analyzed data from 86 countries comparing the Total Cholesterol and Risk of Heart Disease. The graph on the next page shows the results.

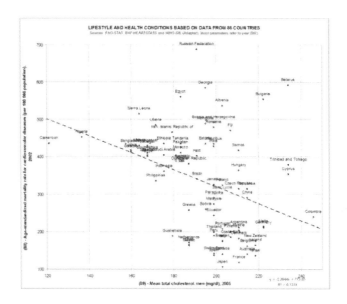

You don't need to be a scientist to see the lack of association. Interestingly, it's quite easy to draw an association in the other direction – in favor of Higher Cholesterol.

The other notable research is from the Lyon Diet Heart Study, which attempted to lower heart disease risk using a diet-intervention instead of drugs (statins) on individuals who had already experienced 1 heart attack. Since saturated fat was the alleged contributor to heart disease at the time, one group was put on a low-fat diet while the other group was told to follow a low carbohydrate diet with no restriction on fat.

In only 6 weeks, the group on the low-carb plan had cut their mortality risk in half (down 56%), and reduced their heart disease risk by 72%!

That being said, the most intriguing part was that Cholesterol levels did not move! If cholesterol levels determine heart disease risk, how is it possible to lower your risk of heart disease by 72% with no reduction in cholesterol?

The reality is, half the people with heart disease have low cholesterol, and half the people with high cholesterol have perfectly healthy hearts.

> Cholesterol has NO ASSOCIATION with heart disease, and study after study will continue to prove this.

However, as long as there's billions of dollars riding on the alternative, we will likely continue to be sheltered from it.

Dietary Cholesterol Does NOT = Blood Cholesterol

Somewhere along the line the assumption was made that the cholesterol you eat raises the cholesterol in your blood. Perhaps it has something to do with the foods highest in cholesterol also being high in saturated fat. It was demonstrated as early as 1937 that dietary cholesterol has very little effect on blood cholesterol, and this fact has never been refuted. However, many still believe that an egg white omelet is 'healthier' for them than eating the yolk.

Limiting foods with saturated fat and cholesterol in our diet in an attempt to lower caloric intake and risk of heart disease is a huge mistake. Other than accomplishing no change in blood cholesterol, it puts our long-term health at risk. Our cells, especially those in the brain, require new cholesterol and essential fats for proper functioning.

68

We utilize 1200-1800mg of new cholesterol every day; which adds stability to membranes, and supports the proper synthesis of hormones.

The Framingham Study from Harvard University Medical School is a perfect example of blood cholesterol remaining unaffected by cholesterol ingestion. Despite dietary intakes that varied by as much as 400mg, the researchers found very similar blood cholesterol levels:

	Cholesterol Intake	Below Median Intake	Above Median Intake
	mg/day	mmol/l	mmol/l
Men	704 ± 220.9	6.16	6.16
Women	492 ± 170.0	6.37	6.26

In fact:

80% of the individuals from the Framingham Study that went on to develop heart disease had the same total cholesterol as those that didn't.

Similarly, the popular Tecumseh Study of 1976 looked at dietary cholesterol intake and total blood cholesterol levels and concluded that:

Less dietary cholesterol produced higher blood cholesterol levels.

The most impactful research study was the Multiple Risk Factor Intervention Trial (MR FIT) from 1982 that took over 360,000 participants and spent $115 Million. The experiment had participants reduce their dietary cholesterol intake by 42% and 28%. Not only was there no reduction in heart disease risk, but blood cholesterol levels barely moved!

Cholesterol = Beneficial NOT Harmful

When we eat more cholesterol our body simply manufactures less or absorbs more. By getting adequate amounts in our diet, we either give our liver a break from assisting in cholesterol manufacturing or we get more of the substance that acts as a building block for cell membranes and a precursor for important hormones (vitamin D, testosterone, androgen). Cholesterol also provides fuel to neurons that can't generate cholesterol on their own.

The biggest benefit from cholesterol is seen in the brain, as it contains 25% of the total cholesterol in the body. It is an antioxidant that supports cell membranes and facilitates communication and transmission of key nutrients and hormones. This is likely why we see cholesterol levels naturally increasing as we age to provide additional protection and nourishment for the brain.

Researchers at Boston University took 789 men and 1,105 women to test for a relationship between total cholesterol and cognitive performance - verbal fluency, attention/concentration, and abstract reasoning.

Participants with good cholesterol levels (under 200, according to the current recommendations) performed poorly compared to those with levels regarded as 'high' (200-239) and 'very high' (>240).

Likewise, a report from the National Institute of Health found the elders that do not have dementia or Alzheimer's had better memory function with HIGHER levels of cholesterol. The researchers write:

"It is possible that individuals who survived beyond age eighty-five, especially those with high cholesterol, may be more robust."

Lower Cholesterol = Bad

Given all the support that cholesterol provides, I suppose it's not surprising that scientists are finding a deficiency in cholesterol and fat in diseased brains. Research is also suggesting an increased risk of neurological disorders with lower cholesterol levels.

A 2008 study from the journal Movement Disorders reported a 350% increased risk of Parkinson's Disease in participants with the lowest cholesterol.

Likewise, in the American Journal of Epidemiology in 2006, researchers from the Netherlands proved that higher levels of total cholesterol were associated with a decreased risk of Parkinson's. Various research studies have also determined a correlation between low cholesterol and depression:

Scientists in a 1993 journal in the Lancet finding a 300% greater risk in the group with the lowest cholesterol, compared to the group with the highest.

71

Research from Sweden in 1997, and the Netherlands in 2000, came to the same conclusion, in both men and women. And sadly, a 2008 report in the Journal of Clinical Psychiatry found that:

> Those with a total cholesterol under 160, were 200% more likely to attempt suicide.

Although speculative, one could hypothesize that the increase in depression over the last 50 years is associated with our questionable efforts to lower cholesterol.

Low cholesterol has also been linked to disrupted hormones, nutrient deficiencies, and even early death.

> A 2009 study that followed 4,500 U.S. veterans for 15 years, showed that those with low cholesterol had a 7-FOLD increased risk of dying.

This is more than likely because of the protection and support that cholesterol provides for cell membranes. This cell support is potentially why we see associations with low cholesterol and nutrient and hormone deficiencies.

> The average testosterone level in males is down 22% compared to 20 years ago!

Given that cholesterol is a precursor for steroid hormones, an adequate intake of essential fats combined with a cholesterol lowering medication can lead to serious disruption. The steroid hormones help control everything from inflammation and metabolism to immunity and fertility.

> Those on statins are more than twice as likely to have low testosterone.

All jokes aside, should we be surprised that decreased libido is the most common complaint from statin users?

Unfortunately, that's not the worst of it...

Statins = Harmful to Health

Although cholesterol has very little to do with heart disease and having low cholesterol can be detrimental to your health, doctors continue to recommend statins to their patients. In fact, the standards for prescribing this pharmaceutical drug have been adjusted significantly over the last 30 years. Statins used to be recommended for someone with a total cholesterol level of 240 that smoked and was inactive. In the mid 80's, the second two risk factors were removed and doctors were able to prescribe cholesterol-lowering meds to anyone with a level of 200. As it sits today, that number is now 180!

Even worse, is that:

> The American Academy of Pediatrics now suggests prescribes statins to 8 year old children, and recommends screening children as young as 2!

Remember, this is for a drug to lower the thing (cholesterol), that has 'no association' with heart disease. That's been unsuccessful in doing what it was designed to do:

> "The incidence, per capita, of heart failure has more than doubled since cholesterol-lowering statin drugs were introduced in 1987."

The drugs designed to prevent heart disease by lowering cholesterol don't prevent heart disease because the problem is not high cholesterol.

Aside from the over diagnosis and ineffectiveness, a recent review study identified over 900 research papers showing adverse effects from statin use (HMG-CoA reductase), including:

- Suppressed immune system
- Increased cancer risk
- Diabetes
- Liver damage
- Muscle degeneration
- Anemia
- Cataracts
- Neuropathy

Early death may be a possibility too, as a study in the American Journal of Cardiology followed 300 adults, determining that:

> Those taking a statin with the lowest LDL cholesterol levels had the highest mortality and those with the highest LDL cholesterol had the lowest.

Other than low testosterone, the most well-known side effect of statins is memory loss. A senior research scientist at MIT, Dr. Stephanie Seneff, has become world renowned for her work connecting statin use with Alzheimer's. She believes statins handicap the liver's ability to make cholesterol, prevent cells from making important antioxidants (coenzyme Q10), inhibit the transport of fatty acids and antioxidants (via LDL cholesterol,) and cause vitamin D and hormone deficiencies.

Monitor Triglycerides NOT Total Cholesterol

John Gofman, a University of California Medical Student, discovered in 1950 that there were circulating fat-like substances in the blood, called Triglycerides. Ultimately concluding that:

> Total Cholesterol was a dangerously poor predictor for heart disease.

Triglycerides that circulate in blood are created in the liver from excess carbohydrates. The majority of us have never been informed that our carbohydrate intake determines our triglyceride levels. Furthermore, that this marker is a much better predictor for heart disease than Total Cholesterol. As researchers from Harvard Medical School determined:

> Those with High Triglycerides and Low HDL Cholesterol have a 6 times greater risk of heart attack, than those with Low Triglycerides and High HDL Cholesterol.

Ironically, our attempts to lower fat intake to prevent heart disease have contributed to increases in carbohydrate food sources, which has increased triglycerides and put us at a higher risk of heart disease.

Along with the Triglyceride-to-HDL ratio, the most reliable biomarker for determining heart health is the composition of LDL cholesterol particles. Although it's often referred to as 'bad' cholesterol, many are unaware that an adequate amount of LDL cholesterol is necessary to transport cholesterol to the brain.

LDL cholesterol particles are benign when they're big and fluffy, but become dangerous when small and dense.

The second slice of irony is that the consumption of plant and vegetable oils (canola, corn, soybean, safflower) are what morphs your LDL cholesterol particles into the small dense variety. Meaning the saturated fats that we were instructed to replace were substituted with vegetable source fats and oils that raise the 2nd critical biomarker for heart disease!

The high carbohydrate and low-fat recommendations over the last 50 years have raised triglycerides, lowered HDL cholesterol, and converted big fluffy benign LDL cholesterol particles into small dense harmful ones.

In other words, the instruction to restrict animal protein and fat to prevent disease, has led to more disease. Not only because of an increase in high-glycemic grains and starches, but because of the shift from saturated to polyunsaturated fats.

"Man is a food dependent creature. If you do not feed him he will die. Feed him improperly and parts of him will die."

— Emanuel Cheraskin (1916-2001)

Choosing The Wrong Fats

When you think about it, calorie restriction and low-fat eating go hand in hand. Fat has 9 calories per gram, while protein and carbohydrates only have 4. Reduce the food with the most calories, and you will lose weight...

...or at least that's how it's supposed to work:

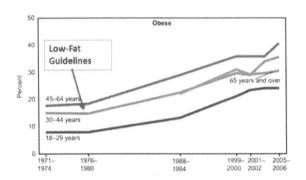

As we've lowered our intake of saturated fat to prevent heart disease and restrict calories to lose weight, obesity has nearly tripled!

Unfortunately, less fat meant more carbohydrates overall, and less animal source foods meant an increase in polyunsaturated vegetable oils (PUFAs). Butter became margarine, coconut oil became canola oil, and more sugar was added. This adjustment was a dream for food producers, as they could now use cheaper oils and get support from the government to do so. Additionally, they could slap a 'low-fat' or 'fat-free' sticker on a bag of chips or box of cookies to give consumers the illusion that their product is healthy.

PUFAs = Heart Disease

Canola oil, soybean oil, cottonseed oil, sunflower oil, safflower oil, peanut oil, and corn oil, are all PUFAs. They're used regularly in restaurants and in the preparation of pre-packaged products because of their affordability. Replacing saturated fat with PUFAs reduces the size of LDL cholesterol particles and decreases HDL (Good) cholesterol. Add the excessive carbohydrates from 'low-calorie' and 'low-fat' whole grains and we've now added elevated Triglycerides to the mix. As we learned in Mistake #4, Triglycerides and small dense LDL particles are the biggest risk factors for heart disease.

In an attempt to eliminate the one-thing we were misled to believe was causing heart disease (saturated fat) we introduced a detrimental alternative.

A 2004 study from the Harvard School of Public Health studied fat intake and it's impact on atherosclerosis (narrowing of the arteries). The researchers concluded that:

> Those who ate the most PUFAs experienced the worst progression, while those eating the highest amount of saturated fat reversed the atherosclerosis!

The high-incidence of heart disease in India we spoke about earlier, is largely because of a switch from saturated fats like coconut oil and ghee (clarified butter) to PUFA alternatives like peanut, safflower, sesame, and soybean oils.

Likewise, a 1993 study in the Lancet showed that a switch from Butter to Margarine increases heart disease:

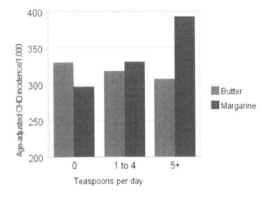

Fats from animal sources are better for our health and body composition, and should be recommended not avoided or replaced. These are the same fats we've relied on for over a million years to support our body and brain with the essentials.

PUFAs = Oxidation & Inflammation

The biggest problem with PUFAs is that they're very unstable and especially susceptible to heat, light, and oxygen. Even though polyunsaturated fats are commonly used for cooking, this is potentially the worst use for them as they oxidize under heat and form free radicals.

A free radical is a molecule with an unpaired electron that grabs an electron from a healthy atom. This not only inflicts damage on the cell where the electron was taken from, but it creates a chain reaction of unpaired molecules.

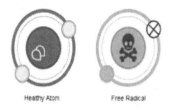

Healthy Atom   Free Radical

The process continues until an electron is taken from a molecule that either 1) changes the cell it's in, or 2) destroys it. This is especially harmful, if that altered molecule is an LDL cholesterol particle (causing heart disease), or a DNA strand (causing aging and cancer).

> The 'free radical theory of aging' hypothesis that cells age because of oxidative stress brought on by having more free radicals present in our body than antioxidants.

Basically, PUFAs cause the problem that antioxidants are supposed to reduce. Saturated fats, on the other hand, are more stable because they have no un-paired electrons. This makes them more resistant to oxidation, and therefore less likely to cause free radical damage.

The 2nd problem with PUFAs is that they're high in Omega-6 fatty acids. As you'll discover in *Live It NOT Diet!*, maintaining a favorable ratio of omega-6:omega-3 is extremely important to your health and longevity as it determines your level of inflammation. Omega-6's fats are pro-inflammatory, which means they cause inflammation, while omega-3 PUFAs like fish oil are anti-inflammatory. When there's more omega-6s than omega-3s, it leads to inflammation. Although there is a healthy intake of omega-6 fats, the replacement of saturated fats with plant and seed oils has created a severely imbalanced ratio. When experienced chronically (as is unfortunately the case for many), this imbalance raises ones risk of developing a degenerative disease considerably. Take a look at the increase in the average omega 6:3 ratio since 1930:

- 8:1 from 1930-1935
- 10:1 from 1935-1985
- 12:1 in 1985 alone
- 25:1 in 2009!

The 6:3 ratio remained relatively consistent for 55 years, and then more than doubled in the next 25. Coincidently, this was over the same 25-year period when we stepped away from saturated fats, and stocked up on polyunsaturated replacements.

This information becomes more devastating when you realize that a healthy ratio is 2:1, and:

Our hunter-gatherer ancestors maintained a 6:3 ratio of 1:1!

We'll talk more on the importance of controlling inflammation and how to balance your omega 6:3 ratio in *Live It NOT Diet!*, but for now it's critical that you recognize the detrimental effect of replacing saturated fats with plant oils. By consuming excess omega-6 polyunsaturated fats, which promote oxidation and inflammation, you increase your risk of nearly every degenerative disease – Parkinson's, cancer, diabetes, Alzheimer's, cardiovascular disease...the list goes on.

Trans-Fats = Hydrogenated PUFAs

The government's support to replace saturated fats with polyunsaturated fats has given marketing agencies the ability to say things like:

'Margarine has 80% less saturated fat than butter, which helps lower your risk of heart disease.'

As I hope you now understand:
- Less saturated fat is not a benefit
- This does not lower your risk of heart disease (it raises it!)

In fact, margarine and other vegetable oils that have been hydrogenated (like shortening) are the worst type of fat. You likely recognize these synthetic fats by their more common name, Trans-Fats. The hydrogenation process to make plant and seed oils solid at room temperature is what morphs them into trans-fats.

86

Ironically, the reason this process was created was to give these oils the same consistency as butter.

Trans-fats are associated with causing severe health issues, specifically an increase in inflammation and elevated risk of heart disease.

> A review of the Nurses Healthy Study determined that just four teaspoons of margarine per day increases cardiovascular disease by 66%!

Unlike saturated fats, which are beneficial to our heart health by raising good (HDL) cholesterol and decreasing small dense (LDL) cholesterol particles, trans-fats do the opposite. Well-respected Harvard researcher, Walter Willet, believes that because of their effect on stroke and heart disease risk, trans-fats could be responsible for nearly 30,000 premature deaths.

> The studies showing a correlation with fat and heart disease use trans fats, not saturated fat.

Other than heart-disease, a small amount of daily trans-fat intake (<2g/day) has been linked to insulin resistance, diabetes, obesity, depression, brain deterioration, oxidative stress, poor cognition, cancer, and increased body pain. Trans-fats have even been linked to aggression and mental decline, which researchers believe is due to inflammation impeding the brain from experiencing the protective and anti-inflammatory effects from omega-3's. Shockingly, most North Americans are unknowingly consuming 3-4g of trans-fats per day as:

The FDA allows companies to include a 'trans-fat free' statement on their product if there's less than 0.5g of trans-fats in it.

Animal Trans-Fats Are Not The Problem

Despite everything you've just learned, I know what you're thinking:

"I'm seeing current research that still blames Red Meat for heart disease, and cancer. What gives?"

Despite the continued practice of citing flawed research, analyzing insignificant biomarkers, and assuming that eating animal foods means cheeseburgers and pizza, there's commonly no clear distinction between animal trans-fat and vegetable source trans-fat. There is an unfair assumption that trans-fatty acids in animal foods are the same as those produced by the hydrogenation of vegetable oils. One is manufactured in a laboratory and the other is naturally occurring, but researchers regularly perform experiments treating the 2 very different substances as equal. The reality is:

Heart disease is only linked to trans-fat from hydrogenated vegetable oils, NOT from naturally occurring trans fats in meat and dairy products.

Similar unwarranted advice comes from research that makes no clear division between linoleic acid from plant source fats, and linoleic acid from animal fats. The consumption of linoleic acid from vegetable oils (LA) is linked to tumor growth, specifically in the breast. While the linoleic acid found in the fat of animals, conjugated linoleic acid (CLA), has been proven effective at preventing cancer, specifically reducing the risk of breast, colon, and skin cancer.

> The linoleic acid (LA) in vegetable oils promotes cancer, while conjugated linoleic acid (CLA) prevents cancer.

Unfortunately, the general public is rarely informed of this VERY important distinction.

"The lower limit of dietary carbohydrate compatible with life is zero, provided that adequate amounts of protein and fat are consumed."

— Institute of Medicine (IOM)

Believing Carbohydrates Are Essential

The typical reasoning for prioritizing carbohydrates is that we need them for energy. For whatever reason, we've all been trained to respond to any mention of cutting carbs with this rehearsed answer. Perhaps our parents said it, we subconsciously heard it in an advertisement, or maybe we took a look at the government food pyramid.

The reasoning is almost laughable when you learn that our primal ancestors averaged less than 80g of carbohydrates per day. Somehow the guy or girl that drives a car to their desk job everyday 'needs' more carbohydrates than someone that walks 5 miles a day, hunts and gathers all their food, climbs trees to escape predators, and physically builds their own shelter (insert sarcasm).

The reality is:

> There is no dietary requirement for carbohydrates.

If absolutely necessary, our body can synthesize any necessary carbohydrate structures from protein and fat. Carbohydrates provide no essential component, and supply none of the elements necessary to build or repair tissue in the body. If we are ever desperate for energy, our body is perfectly capable of making it's own glucose through gluconeogenesis – the process of generating glucose from non-carbohydrate food sources. In fact, the size of our non-carb fuel tank is significantly larger than any ingested or stored carbohydrates could ever provide.

ALL Carbohydrates Become Sugar

The other basic nutritional science the majority of the population fails to recognize, or understand, is that:

EVERY carbohydrate ingested becomes glucose.

Either immediately in the stomach, or eventually in the liver. I won't get into the boring specifics of the different carbohydrate options, but essentially you're looking at monosaccharide's, disaccharides, and polysaccharides. Any guesses what saccharide means…?

....*Sugar!*

What about polysaccharide…?

Many Sugars!!

Regardless of mono, di, or poly, all carbohydrates are eventually absorbed as glucose (or fructose) and thus trigger the same response as sugar.

94

Instead of seeing foods like this:

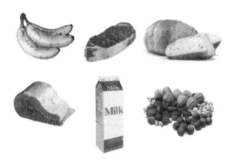

You need to start seeing foods like this:

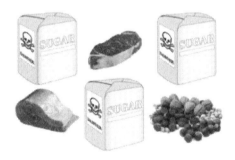

If you're anything like most North Americans, you are unknowingly filling up on foods high in sugar. And I don't just mean candy and sugar in your coffee; I mean cereal for breakfast, a sandwich for lunch, rice or pasta for dinner, and popcorn in front of the t.v. Sadly, our government has us convinced we're being 'healthy,' or making a 'wise choice' when we consume 6-11 servings of grains per day. The reality is:

As you'll soon learn, this is one of the driving forces behind the ridiculous rates of obesity, diabetes, and heart disease.

Another common misconception is that our brain can only function on glucose and requires 120 grams of it per day. Although the 120g requirement is accurate, assuming that this glucose can only be obtained from dietary carbohydrates is where the disconnect lies. Since brain performance is top priority in the hierarchy of importance, our body is quite capable of creating it's own glucose. One of the ways this is accomplished is by breaking down previously stored fat.

Excess Carbohydrates = Fat Storage

Fat is our premium energy source that's readily available to be burned as fuel. The problem is, when we eat excess carbohydrates consistently we never tap into this alternative fuel source, and thus never burn fat. I've found that the easiest way to understand this concept is to think of the body as having 3 empty cups:

- Cup 1 = Glucose to burn immediately for fuel
- Cup 2 = Glycogen to burn if Cup 1 empty (& for exercise)
- Cup 3 = Stored Fat to burn if Cup 1 & 2 empty

Once Cup 1 & 2 are full, any excess carbohydrates are converted to fat in the liver, and either:

- Sent to the bloodstream as circulating fat (triglycerides)
- Stored as body fat (Cup 3)

The greater the excess in carbohydrates, the higher the production of triglycerides and storage of body fat. For example, a 1971 study from the American Journal of Clinical Nutrition put three groups on 1,800 calorie diets that differed only in carbohydrate content.

Protein intake was equivalent in all 3 groups at 115g, but carbohydrates were either 30g, 60g, or 104g per day.

After 9 weeks, fat loss was 15.4, 10.8, and 8.9kg, respectively.

The only way to effectively tap into our fat reserves, while still maintaining our health and nourishing our bodies with essential nutrients, is to lower our carbohydrate intake (empty cups 1&2). The other way to empty those cups is to simply not eat, but then we're burning muscle and putting our long-term health at risk. As I've illustrated, a lack of nutritionally dense calories will lead to malnourishment, hormone disruption, and degeneration. Conversely, by eliminating the 1 macronutrient not required in the diet we burn strictly fat without sacrificing our health.

Excess Carbohydrates = Insulin Resistance

If you look at evolution and the Feast & Famine lifestyle of our ancestors, it becomes easier to understand why we store excess sugar as glycogen and fat (Cup 2&3). Before drive-thrus and fridges, we would go very long periods without food. An extremely important feature should we need to function when food is scarce, but perhaps not as useful when food is consistently available.

When we consume food, our blood sugar rises. This sugar feeds any immediate energy needs, and insulin is secreted to distribute the rest into carbohydrate storage (glycogen) or fat storage (body fat) for future use.

> Insulin is the hormone secreted by our pancreas to help us store glucose for later use.

Although this is an important mechanism to maintain blood sugar homeostasis and store energy for later, when insulin is chronically secreted our storage cells start to become less receptive. The cells already have an adequate supply of glucose, yet insulin continues to attempt to push more in to ensure blood sugar levels are stabilized. Over time the cells either reduce the number of available sites for absorption or turn off completely. When cells no longer respond to insulin, any glucose we consume is more likely to be stored as fat. Meaning even if there is an energy deficit inside the cells, they don't have the receptors to absorb the fuel. Therefore, the daily overconsumption of carbohydrates not only increases the likelihood of glucose converting to fat, but it worsens the responsiveness of our cells to insulin.

> The more comfortable our bodies get with daily sugar consumption the more receptor sites we lose, and the closer we get to insulin resistance (or carbohydrate intolerance).

The more resistant your cells are to insulin, the higher the likelihood that what you eat will become fat instead of muscle. Even after exercise, when we would normally accept large amounts of glucose to store as muscle glycogen (for future use), the cells are unable to absorb carbohydrates. Sadly, this resistance

98

also means amino acids (from protein) and other essentials have difficulty reaching the cells. Making it more difficult to build muscle, in addition to the increased likelihood of storing fat.

In essence, consuming excess carbohydrates is increasing fat storage and decreasing fat burning, along with compounding the rate of each. Aside from the health implications we'll discuss next, many forget to acknowledge that having extra body fat is a risk factor in itself:

> "An increase of one unit of BMI (Body Mass Index) increases the risk of developing heart failure by an average of 20 per cent."

Excess Carbohydrates = Degenerative Disease

When insulin struggles to find somewhere to put excess glucose because of insulin resistant cells, blood sugar remains elevated longer than usual. Aside from causing inflammation, chronically elevated blood sugar (hyperglycemia) is associated with an increased risk of cancer, heart disease, neurological disorders (like Parkinson's and Alzheimer's) and early death.

Excess sugar in the blood also goes through a binding process with proteins and lipids (fats) to form something called AGEs (Advanced Glycation End Products). When glucose attaches to proteins to form AGEs, it gum up arteries and capillaries, and damages DNA, enzymes, and receptor sites. Australian researchers determined in 2004 that:

> AGEs produce a 50-fold increase in free radical production, which accelerates aging and increases ones risk of the same degenerative diseases associated with insulin resistance.

Despite claims favoring a high-fiber plant-based diet to prevent cancer, there's plenty of evidence suggesting otherwise. Dating as far back as 1843, an increase in whole-grain and carbohydrate consumption is highly correlated with an increased risk of cancer. More recently, two studies from Italy tested the relationship between starch intake and breast and prostate cancer. The first study took 1294 men with confirmed prostate cancer, and 1451 men without. It was determined that:

> Men who consumed the most starch had a 1.4 times higher risk of prostate cancer than those consuming the least.

The second study, from the Universita Degli Studi Di Milano, analyzed dietary habits of 2569 women with breast cancer and 3413 women without from 1991-1999. The results were incredible:

> Animal products reduced breast cancer risk by 26%, while the starch-rich diet increased it by 34%!

"Ads are what we know about the world around us."

— James Twitchell

Falling For The Fiber Fallacy

We naturally associate fiber with increasing the speed of digestion. Generally, one thinks that the longer food is in our gut, the higher likelihood that toxins and harmful bacteria will be absorbed and cause damage. The picture you're likely envisioning becomes increasingly prominent when the food sitting in your colon is meat. Not only is animal protein digested slower to begin with, but when we think of harmful bacteria and toxins we generally think of decaying meat. Add the processed, factory-farmed, GMO crop fed, antibiotic pumped meat we wrongfully assume is all that's available, and you get a pretty accurate picture of what a lack of fiber can do…supposedly.

You've already learned that 'Not All Meat is Created Equal,' so the negative vision can be partially eliminated, but there's still a disconnect for most in understanding why slower digestion is not necessarily a bad thing. The reason we all believe we need fiber, and can easily envision the harmful effects of slow digestion, is because it's been driven into our heads for the last 50 years!

The Fiber Fallacy

North Americans were first instructed to eat more fiber after research surfaced from Dr. Denis Burkitt and Dr. Hugh Trowell in the early 70's. They were studying the associations between diet and health status and wanted to determine why the diseases plaguing the Western World were not affecting secluded tribes in Africa. According to their observations, lower colon cancer and heart disease in the African's were attributed to a higher fiber intake. Burkitt and Trowell supplied evidence that the indigestible roughage (fiber) North Americans were removing from their food was providing additional health benefits to the tribesmen. Similar to your vision from earlier, the research suggested that this fiber was increasing digestive flow and preventing the absorption of toxins for the Africans. Very much like the way the 'lipid hypothesis' became a common household recommendation (despite insignificant evidence), this high-fiber hypothesis quickly fast-tracked to fact.

The main reason Burkitt's work was (and is) so believable is that it aligns perfectly with Ancel Keys theory that saturated fat causes heart disease. The world was already leaning towards replacing animal fat and protein with low-fat whole grains to prevent heart disease, and Burkitt's so-called proof helped them make the leap. In reality, Burkitt's work was just as fraudulent as Keys. He conveniently withheld research on African tribes that had low rates of cancer and heart disease, while consuming very little fiber (if any) For instance:

> The Masai in Kenya and Tanzania are virtually disease free, while eating predominantly animal foods with a great deal of fat and an extremely low amount of fiber.

Additionally, the tribes that were consuming small amounts of grains were putting them through intensive fermentation and preparation methods that actually REMOVED the indigestible fiber Burkitt was promoting.

Realistically, there's more than fiber to consider when analyzing secluded populations and comparing them to Western culture. In North America, we are (generally) less active, experience different stress (chronic instead of acute), and deal with more toxins on a daily basis. If you compare a protected group like the Mormons, that eats a low-fiber diet by government standards (less than 25g), their colon cancer and mortality rate is just as low as the tribesmen.

High Fiber Does NOT Lower Disease Risk

Aside from the holes in Burkitt and Trowell's work, there's ample evidence indicating no correlation between dietary fiber and cancer risk. For instance, a 1999 study on 89,000 U.S. Nurses published in the New England Journal of Medicine states:

> "Our data do not support the existence of an important protective effect of dietary fiber against colorectal cancer or adenoma."

With respect to heart disease, companies manufacturing products with whole grains love to promote their products for 'lowering cholesterol,' and being 'heart healthy.' In actuality, there is no proven association between fiber intake and heart disease. The

107

only evidence producing a positive correlation attributed the lower risk to a 'slight' decrease in total cholesterol. As we've discussed, this could be more of a detriment than a benefit; especially if the drop is accredited to a reduction in HDL cholesterol. Unfortunately, consumer products high in whole-grains run with these insignificant findings and use statements in their marketing that continue to mislead the general public:

> *"Foods high in fiber and low in saturated fat reduce the risk of heart disease and certain cancers."*

Meanwhile, when you look at the long-term effects of eating more fiber, research points to an increased mortality rate and a higher risk of heart attack. For example, the DART study from 1989 found that:

> The group eating twice as much fiber ended up with a 23% greater risk of heart attack, and a 27% increased risk of dying.

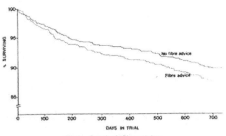

Fig 3—Survival: fibre advice.

This research is especially significant because it tests high-fiber intake over an extended time period. Most research pointing to positive health outcomes from a high fiber diet have been across short timelines; which isn't surprising. When you add indigestible

108

fiber to a poor diet, individuals absorb less of the toxic garbage they're eating, and consume less overall because of the perceived 'fullness' that fiber provides. Although this may produce short-term relief, the long-term impact is negative. As we will discuss next, this is likely the result of damaged intestinal health, chronic inflammation, and poor nutrient absorption.

Whole Grains = Inflammation

The misconceptions surrounding whole grains have been so strong for so long that I often hear this response:

> *"Wheat and crops have been consumed for 100's of years. I've eaten them, my parents ate them, and their parents ate them, and we all survived just fine."*

They may have survived, but how many died of heart disease or cancer?

How many developed Alzheimer's, or were confined to a wheelchair or bed?

Prior to the introduction of whole grains, we lived without many of the degenerative diseases that have unfortunately become common in today's world. Similar to the points made in the saturated fat section, agriculture and modern food processing techniques are not old, they're extremely young:

> "Physicians and nutritionists are increasingly convinced that the dietary habits adopted by Western society over the past 100 years make an important etiologic contribution to coronary heart disease, hypertension, diabetes, and some types of cancer. These conditions have emerged as dominant health problems only in the past century

> and are virtually unknown among the few surviving hunter-gatherer populations whose way of life and eating habits most closely resemble pre-agricultural human beings."

Just because they've been around since you were a baby, doesn't mean they are necessary or healthy.

The most eye-opening study is one comparing low-carbohydrate diets with and without grains on diabetic and pre-diabetic volunteers. After 12 weeks, both groups lost fat and improved their blood sugar, but:

> The grain-free group lost 70% more body fat and were at non-diabetic blood sugar levels at the end of the study.

Other than 'many sugars,' grains (whole or not) contain foreign proteins and natural defenses that induce inflammation. Gluten, found in wheat and other grains, is the most common offender. Regardless of whether there's an obvious allergic reaction (like celiac disease), someone can still experience an immune response to gluten. Several well-respected researchers have suggested that tens of millions of Americans experience this immunogenic response, knowingly or not. After consuming wheat, the immune system releases cytokines because it detects gluten as a foreign substance; and this causes inflammation. Unfortunately for many, this immunogenic reaction goes unnoticed, and it becomes less and less detectable every time the inflammatory food is consumed. The signaling from their digestive system turned off a long time ago, and they may not experience any obvious symptoms until there's a more serious problem.

Big Jimbo with the iron stomach, who can eat 12 hot dog, d drink 10 beers and feel fine, is likely in worse shape on the inside than his outside leads on.

Sadly, it's not just intolerances to immunogenic foods in specific individuals, as all grains are suspected to cause a certain level of inflammation. Whole grains and their flour counterparts are classified as acellular carbohydrates, which produce an unfriendly bacteria in our gut that triggers an inflammatory response. Conversely, fruits and vegetables are cellular carbohydrates that stimulate beneficial bacteria without inflammation. This difference in carbohydrate type is so impactful that groups like the Kitavan Islanders of Oceania can get away with eating a diet as high as 60-70% carbohydrate because they rely solely on cellular sources.

When acellular carbohydrates are introduced to tribes like the Kitavan (even in very small amounts) it produces extreme inflammation and sensitivity.

Aside from being a major contributor to most degenerative diseases (cancer, Alzheimer's, heart disease, etc.), inflammation specific to the gut appears to predict obesity. DIABESITY (obesity + diabetes) caused by chronic inflammation has been strongly correlated with the negative effects of circulating LPS (lipo-polysaccharides), in the gastrointestinal tract. These LPS molecules are elevated when the typical high-carbohydrate grain dominant meal is consumed and can lead to the development of leptin resistance.

The more resistant you become to leptin, the longer you stay hungry, and the less fat you burn overall.

Interestingly, researchers suggest that this chronic gut inflammation is heightened when there is a lack of saturated fat in the diet.

Whole Grains = Intestinal Damage & Poor Absorption

The lectins and phytates found in legumes are also present in whole grains. As previously discussed, these plant defenses decrease the absorption of key nutrients and can damage the walls of the intestinal tract. This tissue damage makes us more susceptible to immunogenic reactions and digestive issues.

Although, many believe soaking and cooking eliminates the majority of lectins and phytates from grains and legumes, some contain lectins that are resistant to heat. Furthermore, as I outlined in the section on plant-based proteins, an 18hr soak only removes 50% of phytates.

> Bran contains phytates that harm iron, calcium, magnesium, and zinc absorption.

When someone demonizes meat because of factory-farming and antibiotics, these characteristics can be changed. We have the ability to choose or produce a higher quality, non-toxic product. The same cannot be said for grains and legumes, as these natural defenses are present in all varieties and can't effectively be removed. More importantly, as companies continue to create more-resistant varieties of crops to support greater yields, these defenses will only grow in number and power.

As the quality of our food and the soil it grows in continues to diminish, the proper breakdown and absorption of the remaining nutrients in foods grows in importance. Since all nutrients are absorbed through the walls of our gut, the integrity of our intestinal lining is extremely important.

> David Southgate, one of the world's leading authority's on fiber, suggests that infants, children, and pregnant women that have greater mineral needs should disregard the recommendation to eat more fiber.

Although the standard recommendation is to consume a high fiber diet, full of cereal grains like Bran, this results in damage to our intestinal lining and compromised digestive health.

The digestive damage from lectins becomes increasingly detrimental with frequent consumption. Unfortunately, this is characteristic of the majority of the population who eats some form of grains at every meal. The cereal for breakfast, sandwich for lunch, pasta for dinner regimen we discussed earlier, introduces toxic lectins frequently and continuously. This constant irritation leaves no opportunity for repair, and can result in a higher severity of damage over time. For instance:

> If the intestinal lining is compromised and more lectins are introduced our risk of leptin resistance is elevated.

This is why one has to question whether adding insoluble fiber to 'speed up' transit time is beneficial; especially for someone with a previously damaged gut.

High Fiber = High Carb = High Risk

Aside from inflammation and digestive distress, an increase in whole grains and cereal fibers adds to our daily carbohydrate (sugar) intake. These polysaccharides ('many sugars') generate a blood sugar response as high as table sugar, and result in excess body fat and elevated triglycerides. However, the general public continues to be misled by the government and various medical associations with statements like this (from 2011):

> "Higher intakes of dietary fiber and whole grain also protect against weight gain and type 2 diabetes, and it is possible that part of the potential effect of fiber intake is mediated through improved weight control and reduced insulin resistance, although these may not be the main mechanisms."

The reality is, insulin resistance is a bigger risk factor for colon cancer; and elevated triglycerides and excess body fat are better predictors of heart disease. The addition of high-fiber whole grains doesn't improve these factors, it makes them worse.

"The more people that believe it's true, the more likely they are to repeat it, and thus the more likely you are to hear it. This is how inaccurate information can create a bandwagon effect, leading quickly to a broad, but mistaken, consensus."

— Barry Schwartz, The Paradox of Choice

Thinking Protein Causes Health Problems

The eating habits we thrived on for millions of years had nearly 4 times the protein the average North American consumes now. Yet, in 2001 The American Heart Association made the following statement:

> "Individuals who follow these [high-protein] diets are at risk for ... potential cardiac, renal, bone, and liver abnormalities overall."

Such a statement is extremely misleading to the public, as there is no convincing evidence to support such a claim. In fact, the research on higher protein diets suggests the exact opposite.

High Protein Does NOT = Kidney Damage

I can't tell you the number of times I've been in a discussion where someone states:

> *"High protein diets cause kidney damage."*

It's almost as if we were all born with an instruction manual that reads:

- Dietary Cholesterol = Heart Disease
- Cut Calories to Lose Weight
- Red Meat = Cancer
- Eat Whole Grains for Fiber
- High-Protein Causes Kidney Damage

The research most are referring to was a *Nurses Health Study* that followed approximately 1600 female participants for 11 years; and ultimately concluded that a high-protein diet causes kidney dysfunction. What the media failed to communicate was that the participants experiencing the damage had <u>pre-existing kidney damage</u> In other words, those with bad kidneys can compromise function of those kidneys by eating a high protein diet. That's like saying:

Someone with an injured shoulder can compromise shoulder function by lifting weights

Or:

A guy with a broken foot can compromise his recovery by jumping up and down.

One of the kidneys main functions is to process the waste products from the food we eat. Eating a high protein diet can increase the filtration work from the kidneys (hyperfiltration), but this is:

"A perfectly normal adaptive mechanism well within the functional limits of a healthy kidney."

In the Nurse's Health Study, those with healthy kidneys did not experience disrupted functionality and many did not even enter a state of hyperfiltration. Furthermore, there's significant evidence suggesting that an increase in protein consumption and a corresponding state of hyperfiltration produces a favorable adaptation from the kidneys. Over time there's less protein found in the urine, which means greater protein absorption.

Since muscle maintenance and growth is dependent on protein synthesis, hyperfiltration should be considered a benefit.

Other than the misleading conclusions drawn from the *Nurses Health Study*, all research on high protein diets and kidney damage have failed to find a correlation in healthy subjects. Even when protein intake was as high as 2.8g per kg of bodyweight, the kidney remained unharmed. For the record, that's 252g of protein per day for a 200lb man; which is the equivalent of four 12oz steaks or eight chicken breasts.

Clearly we should be ignoring the biased recommendations from uninformed organizations and start listening to conclusions from legitimate research:

"It is clear that protein restriction does not prevent decline in renal function with age, and, in fact, is the major cause of that decline. **A better way to prevent the decline would be to increase protein intake.** There is no reason to restrict protein intake in healthy individuals in order to protect the kidney."

Even for those with renal (kidney) disease, there is no benefit from lowering protein intake. Research recommends an intake of at least 1.4g/kg of bodyweight to maintain proper nitrogen balance, or the equivalent of 127g/day for a 200lb man. Sadly, most come nowhere close to that minimum threshold.

They're too busy filling up on high-fiber whole grains!

High Protein Does NOT = Bone Loss

It's commonly believed that a high protein diet causes bone loss because of research showing a considerable (60mg) excretion of calcium in urine for every 50g increase in protein. Since the majority of calcium is stored in bone, it's easy for one to make this assumption. However, this is far from accurate; and as I'll demonstrate, the opposite is true.

Before I get into the research, lets stop and think about this for a second. Protein helps individuals gain and maintain muscle. Muscle surrounds bone, protecting it from damage and providing strength and stability to the musculoskeletal framework. Muscle loss (atrophy) from a lack of dietary protein is highly correlated with bone loss, and a lack of muscle strength with an increased risk of fracture (usually from falling). It's hard to prevent a fall without the muscles to provide stability and hard to prevent a bone fracture without the protection that muscle provides.

The increased risk of fracture is as high as 3 times greater when muscle loss is present.

Generally, a lack of dietary protein is what causes this loss. Therefore, without looking at the potential for leaching calcium from bone, we know that eating a diet high in protein promotes muscle maintenance, providing strength, stability, and bone protection as we age.

Not surprisingly, the science supports this thinking.

> A high protein diet does not negatively affect overall bone density (it increases it!), and we're more at risk from a lack of protein.

The *Framingham Osteoporosis Study* from the year 2000 looked at 615 men and women over 75 years old, and analyzed daily protein intakes ranging from 14g to 175g. Not only did a higher intake show no correlation with bone loss, but those who ate less protein had more bone loss. Other research has shown similar results.

> A study from 1999 in the American Journal of Clinical Nutrition found that an increase in dietary protein reduces the risk of hip fracture in postmenopausal women.

None of this should come as a surprise. Animal foods are our best source of vitamin D other than the sun, and vitamin D blood levels are directly correlated with our absorption of calcium. Several researchers have even suggested that dietary protein is as critical as calcium and vitamin D in the prevention of osteoporosis. As the *Framingham Osteoporosis Study* put it:

> "Even after controlling for known cofounders including weight loss, women and men with relatively lower protein intake had increased bone loss, suggesting that protein intake is important in maintaining bone loss in elderly persons."

Going back to our discussion from the start, it's unrealistic to think that our ancestral diet containing nearly 4 times the protein we consume now all of a sudden negatively affects our bone health. Clearly, a lack of protein is more of a concern than too much.

Protein is Acidic But NOT Harmful

The acid-ash hypothesis suggests that every time we eat and metabolize food, an acid or alkaline ash is left behind that contributes to our overall pH. When that pH is low or acidic our body must fight to maintain homeostasis, which means adding a base to neutralize the environment. Generally, it's hypothesized that this neutralizer is calcium, which would suggest a loss of calcium and bone from an acidic diet.

It has become common practice to blame animal protein for producing an acidic state, despite bread and cheese being equally acidic:

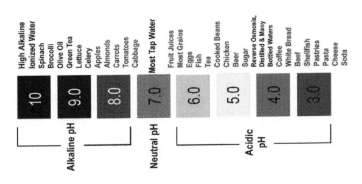

This goes back to my earlier point, that there's an unfortunate assumption that eating animal protein means cheeseburgers and pizza. Before we continue the acid/alkaline discussion, it's important to recognize that swapping meat in favor of high fiber whole grains (as is recommended) does not improve the acidity. Interestingly, if meat was the culprit in producing a low pH one would expect our hunter gatherer ancestors, who derive 35% of their calories from animal protein, to have a net acidic diet. Yet, it's been proven that the pre-agricultural diet is in fact alkaline. This could lead one to assume that perhaps it's the overconsumption of 'other acidic foods' skewing the balance. The point is:

> North Americans are eating an acidic diet whether they include meat or not; especially for those hitting the government recommended 6-11 servings of grains per day.

That being said, an acidic diet is nothing to worry about in the first place. Although additional acid appears to produce more calcium in the urine, research has determined that calcium metabolism is not negatively affected. The acid-ash hypothesis holds true in the sense that there are remnants (acid/ash) left behind after the metabolism of food. However, many fail to acknowledge the important role that the kidneys play in regulating pH.

Bicarbonate ions, found in the blood, are perfectly capable of buffering the acid left behind from protein metabolism. This removes the need for calcium excretion to buffer the acidic environment and maintain homeostasis. These bicarbonate ions act as a neutralizer when acidic foods are ingested and are replaced every time 'new' ones from the kidney are excreted. Meaning, there's calcium, but it's not from bone.

Even though protein is an acid-forming food, it increases the body's ability to excrete acid while improving absorption. Therefore, any excess should be of no concern. In fact:

> Science has determined that a higher protein intake produces positive results in bone health and calcium absorption, and a decreased risk of osteoporosis and fracture.

High Protein Does NOT = Cancer

I hate to pick on vegetarians again, but this is a classic response to justify their decision to avoid meat. I can visualize it now:

> *"Well you know Cancer grows in an acidic environment and meat is vveeerrrryyy acidic."*

Takes bite of bagel with cream cheese, and sip of skinny vanilla latte.

> *"There's tons of research showing that an alkaline diet prevents Cancer growth, and can even remove Cancer Cells."*

First of all, cancer cells can grow in any environment, and most experiments show its growth at normal pH (7.4). Additionally, the body is more tolerant to low pH (acidosis) than high pH (alkalosis), with the lowest survival level at 6.8 (-0.6) compared to the highest survival level at 7.8 (+0.4). Thirdly, most of the theories suggesting an association with cancer and an acidic diet depend on blood and other fluids changing their pH based on the type of food we choose to eat - which is not possible. The pH level of the foods you're eating can effectively alter the acid or alkaline measure of your urine, but cannot adjust the pH of extracellular fluid and blood. Lastly, the ones that do hypothesize that there's a link between dietary acid-forming foods admit that they're only

126

speculating. Any 'expert' understands that once a tumor grows it creates it's own pH.

> *It's not the acidic blood that produces the cancer, it's the cancer that produces the acidic blood.*

Most hate generalizations about any topic, and nutrition is no different. Yet whenever it's suggested that someone increase their animal protein intake, it's met with extreme opposition and unfair generalizations. If anyone knew how uncommon acidosis was in healthy individuals, perhaps they would stop assuming that eating 1 extra piece of meat per day would send them into full blown acid overload and strip their bones of precious calcium. Reaching acidosis from eating an acid-forming diet is nearly impossible.

At the end of the day, it's more than acids and bases. It's food quality and choice, and whole grains are a much bigger concern than meat. Furthermore, if acidity is your biggest worry, perhaps you should know that the acid-load from exercise is a much bigger risk than any potential impact from food.

"While the endurance athlete has a need to maintain a high submaximal intensity for long periods to be successful, the vast majority of athletes, and certainly humans in general, have no need for this type of activity."

— Mark J. Smith, PhD

Exercising To Burn Calories

As mammals, if caloric intake is chronically low (during a diet) or output is chronically high (from exercise) our body naturally seeks homeostasis using a combination of hormones and an adjustment to our metabolic rate. We are able to function on less calories per day because we're storing more and burning less, and attempting to access more calories by elevating our hunger hormones. This is why exercising to burn calories is just as ineffective of an approach to getting fit as attempting to eat less.

The New England Journal of Medicine published research in 2011 on the long-lasting negative physiological effects of a caloric deficit. The reason this research is mentioned here, and not in the calorie restriction section, is because the participants consumed only 550 calories/day. This is characteristic of many extreme weight loss protocols that combine inadequate input (food) with excessive output (exercise). Participants were middle-aged obese men and women that consumed only a 'special' shake and two cups of low-starch vegetables for 10 weeks...

...hmmmm this sounds an awful lot like those MLM Meal-Replacement Shake Diets.

As expected, the men and women lost a lot of weight. However, for the next 42 weeks they gained nearly half the weight back on a maintenance plan that was still restricted. More importantly, their hormone levels remained damaged for an entire year afterwards!

> Leptin decreased, hunger (ghrelin) increased, metabolism slowed, and fat storage was elevated and remained elevated.

Meaning their threshold to gain became significantly lower, and their threshold to burn, higher. As this was only a 10-wk period, one can only imagine the impact from a lifetime of deficits.

When your solution for weight loss and maintenance is caloric reduction, through more exercise or less eating, you fail. The results are short-lived, and unfortunately the damage is long lasting. Consistently fighting hunger is difficult, and trying to push through workouts with no energy is exhausting. As illustrated in Chapter 1, the body senses the caloric imbalance and seeks homeostasis.

> If you won't adjust your energy output (exercise) or energy input (food) to match the demands of your body, your complex hormonal system will do it for you.

Unfortunately, those attempting to lose 'weight' are misled into believing that they need to consume less calories, burn more calories, or do both. Though conventional wisdom will tell them otherwise, they cannot consistently overpower the natural regulators in their body. The reason it seems harder and harder every year, and every time, is because it is!

When your workouts focus on burning calories, your sessions usually revolve around moderate intensity endurance exercise, or cardio.

> *"It must be January, all the treadmills, elipticals, and recumbent bikes are booked up at the gym."*

The reason people select cardio as their method for training because they've bought into the calorie reduction method to losing weight. Just like a calorie restriction eating strategy, this approach will help you lose 'weight' in the short-term provided you can withstand the exhausting workout sessions and extreme battle with hunger. However, as a long-term approach it's not sustainable as our hormones are far too powerful.

Chronic = Elevated Cortisol

Our body possesses the unique ability to adapt quickly to a new challenge. The more we perform the same challenge, the easier it becomes, until it's almost second nature. This phenomenon, known as muscle memory, is especially evident in exercise as weights begin to feel lighter and distances don't seem as far.

In order to experience continuous improvement from exercise, we must consistently change the stimulus or make it more difficult (the overload principle). With resistance training, there's more variables, as the exercise can be altered, weight raised, or repetition and set scheme adjusted. Each minor alteration, even in grip, produces a different stimulus that recruits new muscles that need to adapt. With steady-state aerobic training your body adapts to the stimulus and it requires faster speeds or longer distances to experience the benefits that come with adaptation. Unfortunately, the durations and intensities necessary to experience the 'training effect' initiate higher levels of damaging stress hormones. This results in more fat, less muscle, and a progressive decline in health.

When our body is under stress, the hormone cortisol helps to increase the concentration of glucose in our blood so there's readily available energy for our muscles to utilize. Cortisol secretion is a favorable response when released infrequently and for short periods of time as it helps the body deal with stress. However, when the body is exposed to chronic and consistently elevated cortisol for extended periods of time it can experience unfortunate long-term consequences like cognitive decline, altered immune function, poor digestion, and increased fat storage. Again, this can be related back to the lives of our hunter-gatherer ancestors. They only experienced stress for brief moments in time to run from a predator or chase down prey. This acute, 'fight or flight' response was beneficial, as the cortisol secretion supplied immediate fuel for the brain and muscles to react and function quickly. However, this acute stress is nothing like the daily stress we experience today, and definitely nothing like the stress from prolonged endurance exercise.

The secretion of cortisol starts at the onset of exercise and continues as long as the stressful situation persists. This makes the choice of exercise duration and intensity extremely important. Prolonged endurance training causes the body to release an abundant amount of cortisol. For instance, research from 1976, in the Journal of Applied Physiology showed no increase in cortisol after 10min of exercise (at 75% intensity), but after 30min it doubled. Another study analyzed the cortisol levels in 304 amateur endurance athletes, and the average additional secretion compared to non-endurance athletes (in white) was 42%!

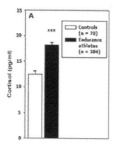

By selecting cardio as your exercise method to getting fit, consistent improvement requires longer distances and higher frequencies. Those who run more kilometers per week, train for more hours, or take part in more competitions over the year consistently exhibit higher cortisol levels.

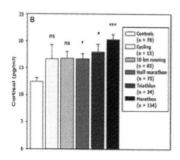

Lifelong endurance athletes are essentially bathing in cortisol and as they continue to push the limits that water gets deeper and deeper.

Intensity plays an equally significant role in determining our stress levels:

> 80% exercise intensity for 1hr raised cortisol, while 40% intensity for 1hr of exercise lowers it.

With an activity like walking, cortisol is removed faster than it can be secreted. However, as individuals looking to get fit we're consistently told to train harder, run further, and burn more calories. The longer cortisol remains elevated, and the more frequently it rises, the more difficult it is to bring it back to homeostasis. When cortisol is chronically elevated, we can't access body fat to burn and we add additional fat to our midsection (visceral or abdominal fat).

Add the stress of your job, kids, finances, and traffic, and is it any wonder we're prone to putting on belly fat?

Chronic Cardio = Testosterone & Muscle Loss

We eat to lose fat, and exercise to build muscle. If your exercise routine revolves around losing, you will ultimately lose...muscle! Muscle memory's effect on endurance training leads to diminishing returns in muscle recruitment and stagnant results from training. More importantly, any attempt to increase the stimulus for additional development will only lead to more cortisol, which produces muscle loss and lowers the hormones responsible for new growth.

136

When cortisol is secreted testosterone is inhibited. Cortisol is catabolic (muscle loss) and testosterone is anabolic (muscle gain), so a negative testosterone to cortisol ratio (T:C) promotes muscle loss. If we select cardio as our method for getting fit, any attempt to improve simply leads to more muscle loss.

A negative T:C ratio translates to a slower metabolic rate, higher risk of degenerative disease (like osteoporosis), and an increased mortality rate.

The other factor contributing to an undesirable T:C ratio is muscle fiber type. The type-1 slow-twitch muscle fibers associated with aerobic athlete (distance runners) favor higher cortisol, while the type-2 fast-twitch muscle fibers associated with anaerobic athletes (sprinters) favor testosterone. Other than genetics, you have a direct impact on the composition of your fiber type by your exercise habits. As illustrated in the chart below, this fiber shift can be significant in only 16 weeks of endurance training at 3-4 sessions per week:

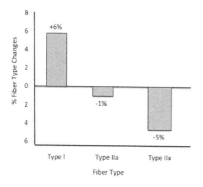

Regular long-distance exercise results in a shift from type-2 to type-1 fibers, which is a continuous process if the activity is frequent and consistent. Interestingly, someone who doesn't exercise (non-athlete) has a better fiber composition than a distance runner.

	% slow (type I)	% fast (type II)
Distance Runner	70-80%	20-30%
Non-Athlete	47-53%	47-53%
Sprinter	25-30%	70-75%

I recognize that women hear 'testosterone' and assume it means they'll turn into a man.

"I just want to get toned."

The reality is, getting toned is a combination of muscle building and fat burning. Unfortunately, prolonged cardio sessions results in the opposite. What most are unaware of, is that testosterone is both anabolic (tissue building) and androgenic (masculine characteristics). Fortunately exercising to build muscle will only lead to increases in anabolic testosterone for women. Although testosterone is generally regarded as a male hormone, maintaining a favorable T:C ratio is just as important for women. Interestingly, research suggests they are more impacted from cortisol secretion during exercise.

Cardio = Inefficient

The actual practice of prolonged aerobic exercise not only favors muscle breakdown, but its time lost when you could have been building muscle. Moderate intensity jogging, cycling, or riding the elliptical for 1-2hrs is extremely time consuming when performed several days a week when equal or better results can be achieved in considerably less time. For example:

> High-intensity sprints produced better fat-loss results and equal performance improvements compared to moderate-intensity jogging, with 1/18th the time commitment.

Most mention doing cardio to improve stamina or endurance capacity, but high-intensity interval training (HIIT) has proven more effective at improving aerobic power, lactate threshold, and Vo2 Max. From an efficiency perspective:

> It makes no sense to spend 1-2hrs on something that can be done in 20min, and without the potential for muscle loss and fat gain.

Half of the time spent running could have been invested in weight-training or interval training producing more metabolically active muscle, burning more fat, raising beneficial hormones (testosterone, GH, IGF-1), and avoiding the accumulation of cortisol. When you workout to build muscle you burn more energy throughout the day, as this new muscle needs additional fuel to operate. Meaning you will burn more without additional exercise.

Aerobic training, on the other hand, does not produce positive changes in muscle and the intensity and duration must continue to increase in order to experience additional burning. Longer distance and higher intensities means more cortisol and muscle loss, and less testosterone. As I'll illustrate next, this stressful environment not only impacts your body composition, but it raises your risk of the various diseases of degeneration.

"If we went out for a run right now and you ran hard... by 60 minutes something starts happening... the free radicals blossom, and it starts burning the heart. It starts searing and inflaming the inside of your coronary arteries."

— Dr. James O'Keefe

Doing Cardio To Stay Healthy

Ask any rehabilitation specialist (physio, chiro, massage therapist), and they'll tell you how detrimental chronic repetitive movements can be on muscles, joints, bones, ligaments, and tendons. At first glance, moderate intensity endurance exercise may seem like it's easier on the body than weight training or interval training, but it's not. The same consistent impact for hours at a time causes hip pain, knee pain, or ankle pain, and overall inflammation. Even worse is that individuals doing this as a weight loss strategy are generally putting higher loads on their ligaments and joints.

Exercising at a slow pace for a long time is extremely unnatural. Our hunter-gatherer ancestors would probably laugh watching us run, bike, or swim for hours to burn calories. Back then, energy was conserved, and you either walked to get somewhere, or you ran really fast to get away from something. Even when hunter-gatherers developed organized hunting, they relied on their brains and other resources to track and trap animals, not chase them around for 3hrs! One could imagine what a huge waste of energy it would be if a 3hr persistent hunt was unsuccessful. Furthermore, recent findings provide evidence that the earliest form of human was not designed to run because the conical shape of the ribcage made it difficult for them to swing their arms.

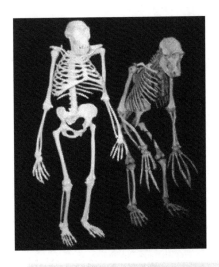

"They probably couldn't run over longer distances, especially as they were unable to swing their arms, which saves energy."

We can even forget the hunter-gatherers for a minute, and take a look at children playing to determine what's 'natural.' When kids are playing outside at the park, they unknowingly move in short bursts followed by ample recovery. Oddly, there was a study done on this exact scenario. Researchers determined that children naturally exercise in intervals, as opposed to moving at a consistent speed.

Looking at the medical records runners, it's not surprising that they're frequently injured. The irony in the term 'stress fracture' is almost laughable when you think of the excess stress one can expect from chronic and prolonged aerobic training.

Cardio Generates Excess Free Radicals

When we hear the word 'cardio,' most of us think of jogging, biking, swimming, or anything that gets your blood pumping at a reasonable rate. As already illustrated, these activities produce negative consequences in body composition by supporting muscle damage as opposed to growth, and fat storage as opposed to removal. When it comes to your long-term health, less muscle and more fat is obviously not favorable. However, the biggest issue with moderate-to-high intensity aerobic exercise is that it results in an overabundance of free radicals.

Our body produces it's own antioxidants to counteract free radicals, and can naturally increase its level to maintain balance or homeostasis. However, if free radicals continuously outnumber antioxidants, damage ensues.

I tend to understand free radical production best, when I think of it like inflammation. Acute inflammation is necessary so that our body can go to work on fixing whatever issue we're encountering that trigged the response (ex: cut on arm). However, when this response is chronic (ex: gut irritation), and out of balance with our anti-inflammatory levels, there is a problem. Similarly, acute and infrequent free radical production is necessary for adequate cell function (like facilitating energy production in mitochondria), but if free radical accumulation is chronic and out of balance with antioxidant levels, there's a problem.

Free radicals are produced during muscle contractions during physical exercise. Nearly every workout type - aerobic or anaerobic, high-intensity or low-intensity, isometric or isokinetic - produces free radicals, but the amount generated varies based on the mode, intensity, and duration of the activity. Some argue that high levels from exercise are beneficial because they increase the body's internal production of antioxidants. Supposedly this promotes higher antioxidant levels to deal with increased amounts of free radicals. However, similar to cortisol, research suggests that problems arise when free-radical production is extremely high (2hr run), or extremely frequent (running 5 days/wk). In this case, instead of continuing to increase its threshold in the presence of elevated free radicals, the cells will become damaged or even destroy themselves to protect the rest of the body.

A model developed in 1992 by M.B. Reid suggests that free radical production is necessary at low levels to preserve normal muscle performance, but higher concentrations produce negative effects. During strenuous exercise free radicals are generated faster than any buffering agent can handle, and this impairs performance and force output. His model implies avoiding full fatigue, favoring moderate free radical accumulation that favors increased performance and promotes a natural antioxidant response in balance with free radical concentrations.

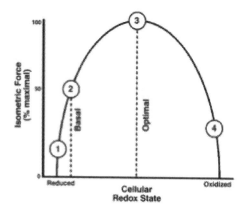

Above the optimal threshold, oxidation outnumbers antioxidants, and thus harmful oxidative stress will prevail - leading to muscle dysfunction and loss, damage to protein, lipids and even DNA.

Cardio Produces Acidic pH

The other potentially harmful substance generated during aerobic exercise is lactic acid. Again, this substance is produced during exercise based on intensity and duration, and is an important consideration as an exercise stressor because it lowers pH. Simply running for a few minutes, drops our normal pH of 7.4 to 7.0. Continuing or repeating the same activity can lower it to 6.8, which is considered the lowest tolerable survival pH.

As we discussed earlier, many mistakenly think that cancer can only grow in an acidic environment and attempt to blame food for that, yet conveniently forget that their 2hr run that same morning puts them in a more harmful state of acidosis (low pH). The buffering systems (to bring pH up) we have built-in to handle an acidic-food are not as effective during exercise. For instance, the kidneys regulate pH after an acidic meal by excreting more or less bicarbonate. Unfortunately, this is an ineffective regulator for dealing with the pH stress from exercise, as it can take several hours to react. Additionally, research that supports correlations between cancer and pH focus on increased acidity (low pH) in blood and other fluids.

> Our diet cannot alter the pH in blood, whereas our exercise habits can.

Large amounts of lactic acid are produced during exercise that's beyond a certain intensity or duration, and this increases oxygen and acidity (lowers pH) inside and outside muscle cells. Accumulation of lactate depends on a balance between production by the working muscles and removal by the liver and other tissues. If exercise is continuous, lactate production persists while removal declines. This lactate build-up not only adds to the stress put on our cells, but:

> Arterial pH disturbance alone has been associated with life-threatening rhythmic disturbances of the heart.

Cardio = Respiratory & Reproductive Damage

One of the reasons endurance exercise is more damaging than other forms of exercise, such as weight training, is because intense oxidation and acidity occurs in all 'active' muscles. For instance, diaphragm muscle is continuously stressed throughout an endurance bout, meaning that free radical and lactate accumulation is consistently produced for the entire 45, 90, or 120min bout.

150

With cardio, the same muscles are experiencing the same high stress and low pH during the entire duration. This concentrated overload is what causes damage, as opposed to a properly designed weight training program that stresses a single muscle or group of muscles for a short period of time followed by ample recovery. Furthermore, most involved in weight training allow ample recovery (72hrs) between muscle groups, as opposed to cardio where it's extremely common to return to the pavement, bike, or pool the very next day!

Specifically, endurance athletes are at a higher risk of upper respiratory tract infection (URTI), similar to what one would experience from over-training or too much stress. Again, there's appears to be a positive correlation with longer durations and higher frequencies:

> 6 times as many runners experience URTIs following marathons compared to non-participating runners.
>
> Runners that run 96km/week or more, had twice the risk of URTI than those doing 32km/week (1/3rd the mileage).

Intensity also plays a factor as walking seems to produce favorable reductions in URTIs:

> Elderly individuals walking 45min 5xWeek reduced infection by 50% compared to sedentary.

The rate of infection appears to be the worst when there's a moderate-to-high intensity (60-80%) combined with a longer duration (90min):

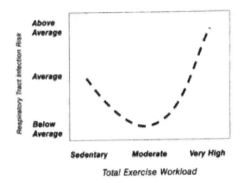

Total Exercise Workload

And it's not just runners!

> One study looking at 24 swimmers, found higher rates of respiratory infection in the well-trained swimmers (56%), compared to the amateurs (12.5%).

Although speculative, this suggests that it's the chronic repetitiveness of the exercise and the cumulative affect on the body that causes the damage. Interestingly, excessive is defined as "training with insufficient rest and variety ."

Asthma and allergies appear to be highly prevalent as well, as one study tested 42 elite runners of which 23 had asthma and 31 asthma like symptoms. Another study from Finland tested 103 athletes with an average age of 23, and reported 16 with asthma, 24 with allergies, and more than half with asthma-like symptoms or exercise-induced asthma.

With respect to reproductive health, amenorrhea (a disruption in menstrual cycle) is highly prevalent in female endurance athletes.

A 1984 study in the American Journal of Sports Medicine, found that 29% of female endurance athletes have amenorrhea.

Researchers point to a 'lack of available calories' as the driving force in producing these unfavorable consequences. Although, it's also suspected that the 'amount' of training is to blame for this elevated risk. Either way, we see similar damage in men:

A 1994 study found that high-mileage male runners have lower sperm counts and motility than low-mileage runners.

Considering the extremely high blood concentration of stress hormones with longer durations and higher intensities, it's not surprising to see the disrupted release of reproductive hormones. The oxidative stress from long distance endurance training produces significant decreases in the size of the reproductive organs, and cortisol has been shown to reduce testosterone and androgen levels.

The other important consideration for those deciding to partake in long-distance running is the increased loss of blood, and the iron that goes with it. Women are already at an extremely high risk of anemia (low iron) because of their monthly blood loss, and low red meat intake in general. Research has identified a clear link between anemia and runners, and the statistics suggest that it's also quite prevalent in males.

Endurance athletes appear to be at a consistent iron deficiency, losing 1.7-2.2g/day while only absorbing 1g/day.

Cardio = Heart Damage

Although the other negatives of selecting cardio to stay healthy have been eye opening, this one tends to sting the most. Mainly, because the reason a lot of people decide to start running or biking is to improve their 'heart health.' One can't help but think of someone out there running their butt off to get in shape or stay healthy, when in fact they're doing more harm than good. As they continue to push the limits and work to strengthen their blood pumping muscle, they actually do the opposite and put their cardiovascular health at risk.

Overtraining is a common mistake many athletes make in preparation for competition, and it appears to be just as common in the general population when they decide it's time to 'get fit.' January 1st roles around and the out of shape guy at work says:

"My goal this year is to run a marathon!"

Although our body physically adapts as best it can during frequent and intense training, many times the damage isn't felt until it's already too late. When it comes to endurance exercise, this is especially true. Our natural defenses endure the consistent mileage increases, and compensate for the elevated intensity until one day our heart shuts down. This can be seen in the cardiovascular health of ultra-endurance athletes, who continuously put their bodies through a pounding. These guys, and girls, aren't just running further than everyone else, they're running more consistently and

154

faster. Most (including me) would like to idolize these individuals as we can't see ourselves doing 1 marathon, let alone 2 in a row on a Saturday afternoon. However, the duration and intensity of exercise has a profound effect on free radical generation; and despite the natural increase in antioxidant protection, that threshold is surpassed and serious damage ensues.

As Dr. James O'Keefe points out, endurance training causes 'structural cardiovascular changes' and 'elevations of cardiac biomarkers' that appear to return to normal in the short term, but as taken on as a regular activity it results in:

> "patchy myocardial fibrosis...an increased susceptibility to atrial and ventricular arrhythmias, coronary artery calcification, diastolic dysfunction, and large-artery wall stiffening."

O'Keefe mentions that it's common to see abnormal results in heart tests for elite level endurance athletes, with as high as a 5-FOLD increase in the prevalence of atrial fibrillation. With ultra endurance athletes, and Cardio Kings and Queens, the damage is especially detrimental as each workout of increased intensity and duration produces more free radicals and considerable damage. One study, from the European Heart Journal looked at marathon runners, triathletes, alpine cyclists, and ultra triathletes, who competed in races lasting 3, 5, 8, and 11hrs respectively.

> Dysfunction in the right ventricle after the race was least in the marathon runners (3hrs), and highest in the ultra triathletes (11hrs).

Although the evidence is still emerging, there's a budding amount of research that frequent long distance endurance training leads to cardiovascular damage and increases heart disease:

- Impaired Cardiac Contractile Function
- Decline in Peak Systolic Tissue Velocity
- Cardio Myocyte Damage
- Myocardial Fibrosis
- Atrial Fibrillation
- Cardiac Arrhythmias
- Poor Left Ventricle Function

These elevations and alterations could be the result of adaptive responses our body goes through in order to deal with the physically taxing and stressful workout. However, it's clear that this adaptation is not favorable in the long-term. One could relate this to our hunter-gatherer ancestors who occasionally had to deal with unique challenges and intense feats of strength that would require an above-average adaptation to survive. Although, just because we can adapt doesn't mean we should; especially on a consistent basis. The resulting heart damage has been witnessed in the early (or near death) of several famous ultra-endurance and marathon runners:

Micah True *(Caballo Blanco) - one of the ultra runners featured in the popular book Born to Run, died in 2012 at 58 years old of Phidippides cardiomyopathy (enlarged heart from chronic excessive endurance exercise!)*

Alberto Salazer – won 3 New York City Marathons and 1 Boston Marathon between 1980 and 1982, had a near fatal heart attack at 49 years of age

156

Jim Fixx - *the man credited for popularizing jogging and author of the best-selling book, The Complete Book of Running, died of a heart attack at 52!*

Cardio = Early Aging?

When the original free radical theory was revisited it evolved into what we now know as the mitochondrial theory of aging. Basically, scientists recognized that damage specific to mitochondrial DNA was responsible for increasing disease risk and shortening lifespan.

> One analysis of skeletal muscle from a 90-year-old man revealed that only 5% of his mitochondrial DNA was full length, while that of a five-year-old boy was almost completely intact.

Telomeres are found at the ends of chromosomes that protect DNA and the length of these tiny caps can determine our rate of aging. Our telomeres shorten during normal cell division, but if they get too short, chromosomes get damaged, cells stop dividing, and our ability to repair tissue is inhibited. Numerous studies have found that short telomeres are associated with older cells and an increased risk of mortality and disease, and longer telomeres are associated with younger cells and a higher resistance to disease. The exact cause of telomere shortening is still up for debate, but the leading hypothesis points to chronic stress. Not only does excess stress cause DNA damage, but it appears to disrupt the enzyme responsible for telomere elongation (telomerase) - meaning any chance of future repair and growth is inhibited.

Exercise is an important consideration because mitochondria produce a fair amount of free radicals during physical activity. We know that the duration and intensity of your workout determines the free radicals produced, and there's a certain threshold at which accumulation overburdens our anti-oxidant defenses. We also know that this damage accumulates over time, making each additional session of equal intensity or duration increasingly harmful. What we haven't discussed, is that our exercise method determines 'where' these free radicals are produced.

With consistent movements lasting more than 60 seconds (aerobic), oxygen is required to produce energy. This oxygen requirement means free radicals are produced within mitochondria. Conversely, short or intermittent (anaerobic) exercise does not require oxygen to produce energy.

> During aerobic exercise, energy production takes place inside mitochondria using oxygen. During anaerobic exercise energy is produced outside mitochondria; as oxygen is not needed.

Since mitochondria are the biggest producers of free radicals, skeletal muscle contains the most mitochondria, and muscle represents the largest organ in the body, this is a BIG problem. Not only because a higher level of free radicals increases the likelihood of cell damage, but because mitochondrial DNA damage appears to predict our lifespan.

> Free radical damage from long and frequent cardio workouts is especially detrimental to cardiac and skeletal muscle, encouraging muscle catabolism and potentially increasing heart disease risk.

Chronically elevated cortisol is nearly as detrimental with respect to disease; as aside from discouraging anabolic hormones, it promotes unnecessary inflammation in the brain, reproductive system, intestinal tract, and heart.

> The elevated inflammatory markers experienced after aerobic exercise are much higher than those tested after alternative forms of exercise.

The other factors producing inflammation are free radicals and chronically elevated insulin. Sadly, both are characteristic of the long distance runner, cycler, or swimmer, who trains too long and too often, and tends to rely heavily on a high-sugar, high-carb diet.

Inflammation and oxidation are two of the biggest factors in determining whether or not you develop a life threatening disease. Both are necessary in acute and infrequent doses for survival, but when experienced chronically, the biological clock starts ticking.
In either case, a balance can be achieved by obtaining more of the reducing agent (anti-inflammatory or antioxidant) or avoiding the promoting agent (inflammation and free radicals). In both instances, it seems more reasonable to avoid the promoting agent – i.e. Cardio!

I know it seems odd for me to be a nutrition and fitness advisor yet I'm openly discouraging endurance exercise. However, much like my philosophy on nutrition, I'm not an advocate of aerobic training because I know there's a better alternative that doesn't come with negative consequences.

Soy is detrimental at over 36g; wheat causes inflammation and digestive distress; so why consume them at all?

Cardio elevates cortisol and lowers testosterone, burns muscle and stores fat, and promotes cell damage through oxidative stress; so why do it at all?

Clearly, there's a safe level of exercise, and frequent cardio sessions for extended periods of time surpass that level. I assure you that your time is better spent building muscle that burns fat, and eating in a way that has you burning fat as fuel instead of sugar. Not only because that's the most efficient use of your time to get the results you desire, but because it gives you the best chance at slowing the aging process...

...instead of unnecessarily accelerating it.

"Everybody is a genius. But if you judge a fish by its ability to climb a tree, it will live it's whole life believing that it is stupid."

— Albert Einstein

So What Now?

The reason I took the time to write this book is because I continue to watch the 'common' approach negatively affect those around me. They usually last about 2 months trying to 'burn calories' on the treadmill, and 'eat less' high-calorie foods; fighting a daily battle with hunger and low energy. Conventional wisdom is leaving them:

OVERWORKED and UNDERFED!

Once they fall off their 'diet' and put more weight on than when they started, they beat themselves up because the universal theory of calories-in vs. calories-out implies that they lack discipline. As I hope I've demonstrated throughout this text:

"You've been hitting the bull's-eye on the wrong target!"

Now that you've read *Eat Meat And Stop Jogging*, you should be aware of the nonsense. You understand why 'everyone else' believes, and 'everyone else' follows bogus advice. The question is, do you want to continue looking, feeling, and living like 'everyone else'?

Take a look around next time you're in public and make note of the body composition of those around you. Individuals in their early 20's with 40% body fat, school children with the physique of a middle-aged stock broker, and baby boomers hobbling around like seniors, from hip fractures, triple-bypasses, and knee surgeries. The reason we look the way we do is because of the food we eat, fitness regimen we follow, and lifestyle choices we make. The misconceptions you just discovered are what most have been attempting to follow for the last 50 years, and where has it landed them?

The question is:

Are you going to sit back and accept that this is the new 'normal,' and we're all destined to be fat and unhealthy?

Or:

Are you ready to open your eyes to a BETTER way of eating, a BETTER way of training, and a BETTER way of living?

Now that you understand the misconceptions that continue to set you up for failure, I can finally introduce *Live It NOT Diet!*

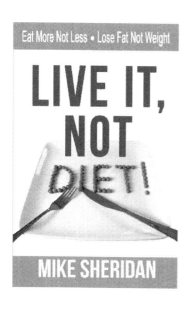

Eat More Not Less • Lose Fat Not Weight

LIVE IT, NOT DIET!

MIKE SHERIDAN

With this unbiased, non-corporately funded program you will achieve the toned, healthy, muscular, sexy physique you've been striving for, and if embraced as a lifestyle, you will maintain your results well into the future. Not only that, but you'll get there without fighting your innate need to eat when you're hungry and until you're full. Never again will you count calories or monitor portion size, feel deprived or weak, or experience the endless yo-yo cycle of losing it and gaining it back.

> My program works for me, and it has worked for 100's of clients - it works because it's sustainable!

Now I can't promise you'll be a fitness model or world class athlete, but I will guarantee:

Weekly Fat Loss WITHOUT Muscle Loss!

In this follow-up text, I tell you what to eat in a way that gives you the ability to dedicate minimal time and effort to 'getting fit' while experiencing amazing results. I introduce you to 14 Principles and progress you across 3 phases until you're presented with the *Live It NOT Diet!* Lifestyle Plan, which has been followed by myself and my clients for years. We eat as much as we want, whenever we want, and never do cardio; while maintaining a lean and healthy physique, and strong body and mind.

The difference between *Live It NOT Diet!* and other approaches, is that it's designed to be embraced as a long-term strategy. I progress you at a comfortable speed, so you're programmed for consistent success. My clients that have followed this plan achieve amazing results, but more importantly they maintain them long after they've gone on their own.

If you're ready for superior and sustainable results while improving your health and longevity, I hope you will JOIN ME and thousands of North Americans in getting lean, and staying lean…for LIFE!

Coach Mike

Live It NOT Diet! Special Offer

In an effort to gather feedback on *Eat Meat And Stop Jogging*, I'm offering $5 off your purchase of *Live It NOT Diet!* I'd love to hear about your experience with the book so that I can continue to improve my message, and the way in which I deliver it.

All you have to do is:
- Share your experience with the book in an Amazon Review
- Copy and paste the link to your review at:
  - http://eatmeatandstopjogging.com/myreview/
- Wait 24hrs for your $5 gift card to arrive by email

If you already purchased *Live It NOT Diet!*, the $5 is still applied to your account so you can save on future purchases.

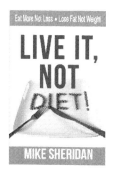

Whether you decide to comment or not, you can access *Live It NOT Diet!* by visiting this link:

http://amazon.com/Live-It-NOT-Diet-Weight/dp/0993745555

About The Author

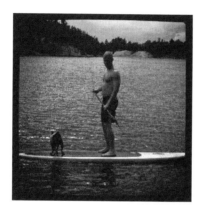

Mike Sheridan is a research-obsessed Nutrition and Fitness Expert on a mission to uncover the backwards advice on what it takes to be healthy and fit. As an aspiring professional football player, Mike's obsession with human performance began at an early age, and directed him towards a career in personal training and nutrition. Although Mike has been able to help a tremendous amount of people transform their body and their life, he has an inherent need to extend his reach and communicate the enormous gap between the scientific evidence and the message to the public. Instead of letting faulty advice continue to negatively affect the health and body composition of those around him, Mike decided to invest his extra energy into relentless self-study. After years of research and nearly a decade of personal practice, Mike shares his knowledge and experience in *Eat Meat And Stop Jogging*.

References

Introduction

Oppenheimer, D. M. 2006. Consequences of erudite vernacular utilized irrespective of necessity: problems with using long words needlessly. Applied Cognitive Psychology 20(2):139-156.

Song, H., et al., 2009. If It's Difficult to Pronounce, It Must Be Risky: Fluency, Familiarity, and Risk Perception. Psychological Science 20(2):135-138.

National Health and Nutrition Examination Survey. 1999. Prevalence of Overweight and Obesity among United States Adults 1999-2002. Hyattsville, MD: National Center for Health Statistics

Cheng D. 2005. Prevalence, predisposition and prevention of type II diabetes. Nutrition & Metabolism 2:29.

Moons, W. G., Mackie, D. M., Garcia-Marques, T. 2009. The impact of repetition-induced familiarity on agreement with weak and strong arguments. Journal of Personality and Social Psychology 96(1):32-44.

Mistake #1

Selye, H. 1955. Stress and disease. Science 122:625-631.

BGM Models (May, 2012). Marie Claire Average Weight Feature. Retrieved From<http://www.bgmmodels.com/marie-claire-average-weight-feature/>

Booth, F., and S. Weeder. 1993. Structural aspects of aging human skeletal muscle. In Musculoskeletal Soft Tissue Aging Impact on Motility, ed. Rosemont, IL: American Academy of Orthopaedic Surgeons

McNaughton, S., Wattanapenpaiboon, N., et al. 2011. An Energy-Dense, Nutrient-Poor Dietary Pattern is Inversely Associated with Bone Health in Women. Journal of Nutrition 141(8), 1516-1523.

Torjesen P. A., Sandnes L. 2004. "Serum testosterone in women as measured by an automated immunoassay and a RIA". Clin. Chem. 50(3):678-9

Southren A. L., et al., 1967. "Mean plasma concentration, metabolic clearance and basal plasma production rates of testosterone in normal young men and women using a constant infusion procedure…". J. Clin. Endocrinol. Metab. 27 (5):686–9

Donnelly, J. E., J. Jakicic, and S. Gunderson. 1991. Diet and body composition: Effect of very low calorie diets and exercise. Sports Medicine 12:237-49.

Foster, G. D., et al. 1990. Controlled trials of the metabolic effects of a very-low calorie diet: short- and long-term effects. American Journal of Clinical Nutrition 51:167-72.

Kekwick, A., and Pawan. G. L. 1957. "Metabolic Study in Human Obesity, with Isocaloric Diets High in Fat, Protein, or Carbohydrate, Metabolism 6:5.

Kekwick A, Pawan G. L. 1956. "Calorie intake in relation to body-weight changes in the obese". Lancet 271 (6935): 155–61.

Bray, G. A., et al., 2012. Effect of Dietary Protein Content on Weight Gain, Energy Expenditure, and Body Composition During Overeating: A Randomized Controlled Trial. JAMA. 307(1):47-55.

Poehlman, E. T. 1989. A review: Exercise and it's influence on resting energy metabolism in man. Medicine and Science in Sports and Exercise 21:515-25.

Nielsen S, et al., 2003. Energy expenditure, sex, and endogenous fuel availability in humans. J Clin Invest 111: 981-988,

Benedict, F. G. et al. 1919. Human Vitality and Efficiency Under Prolonged Restricted Diet. Washington, D.C.: The Carnegie Institute of Washington

Keys, A., et al. 1950. The Biology of Human Starvation, vol. 1. Minneapolis: The University of Minnesota Press.

Passmore, R. 1968. Energy metabolism at various weights. In Metabolism, ed. 344-45.

Welle S and Nair KS. 1990. Relationship of resting metabolic rate to body composition and protein turnover. Am J Physiol Endocrinol Metab 258:E990-E998.

Sumithran, P., Prendergast, L., et al. 2011. Long-Term Persistence of Hormonal Adaptations to Weight Loss. The New England Journal of Medicine 356(17), 1597-1604.

Spiegel, K., et al., 2004. "Brief Communication: Sleep Curtailment in Healthy Young Men is Associated with Decreased Leptin Levels, Elevated Ghrelin Levels, and Increased Hunger and Appetite." Annals of Internal Medicine 141(11):846-50.

Bray, G. A. 1969. Effect of calorie restriction on energy expenditure in obese patients. The Lancet 2:397-98.

Boelsma, E., et al., 2010. Measures of postprandial wellness after single intake of two protein-carbohydrate meals. Appetite. 54(3):456-64.

Leidy, H. J., et al., 2011. Neural Responses to Visual Food Stimuli After a Normal vs. Higher Protein Breakfast in Breakfast-Skipping Teens: A Pilot fMRI Study. Obesity 19(10):2019-2025.

Boelsma, E., et al., 2010. Measures of postprandial wellness after single intake of two protein-carbohydrate meals. Appetite. 54(3):456-64.

Cavadini C, Siega-Riz AM, Popkin BM. 2000. US adolescent food intake trends from 1965 to 1996. Arch Dis Child. 83:18-24.

Christian, J. L., and J. L. Greger. 1994. Nutrition for Living. Red Wood City, CA: Benjaming/Cummings

Tropp J, Markus EJ. 2001. Effect of mild food deprivation on the estrous cycle of rats. Physiol Behav 73: 553–559.;

Hill JW, Elmquist JK, Elias CF. 2008. Hypothalamic pathways linking energy balance and reproduction. Am J Physiol Endocrinol Metab 294:E827–32.

Booth PJ, et al., 1996. Endocrine and metabolic responses to realimentation in feed-restricted prepubertal gilts: associations among gonadotropins, metabolic hormones, glucose, and uteroovarian development. J Anim Sci 74: 840–8.

Quesnel H, et al., 1998. Influence of feed restriction during lactation on gonadotrophic hormones and ovarian development in primiparous sows. J Anim Sci 76: 856–63.

Veldhuis JD, et al. 1993. Amplitude suppression of the pulsatile mode of immunoradiometric luteinizing hormone release in fasting-induced hypoandrogenemia in normal men. J Clin Endocrinol Metab 76:587–93.

Brito LFC, et al. 2007a. Effect of feed restriction during calfhood on serum concentrations of metabolic hormones, gonadotropins, testosterone, and on sexual development in bulls. Reprod 134: 171–181.

Brito LFC, et al. 2007b. Effect of nutrition during calfhood and peripubertal period on serum metabolic hormones, gonadotropins and testosterone concentrations, and on sexual development in bulls. Domest Anim Endocrinol 33: 1–18.

Garthe, Ina. 2012. Changes in Body Composition and Performance in Elite Athletes During A Period with Negative Energy Balance Combined with Strength Training.

Eighth International Conference on Strength Training. Norwegian School of Sports Sciences.

Mistake #2

Cordain, L. "Cereal Grains: Humanity's Double-Edged Sword," World Review of Nutrition and Dietetics 84 (1999): 19-73.

Ingenbleek, Y., McCully, K. 2012. Vegetarianism Produces Subclinical Malnutrition, Hyperhomocysteinemia, and atherogenesis. Nutrition. 28:148-153.

Ross, J. The Diet Cure. (Penguin Books; NY), 1999. 102-113.

Price, W. A. Nutrition and Physical Degeneration. (Keats Publishing; CT.),1989, 256-281.

Groff, J. and S Gropper. Advanced Nutrition and Human Metabolism, Third Edition. (Wadsworth/Thomson Learning; CA.), 1999, 317.

Cooper, C. et al. 1996. Dietary protein and bone mass in women. Calcif Tiss Int, 58:320-5.

Chiu, J. F. et al., 2997. Long-term vegetarian diet and bone mineral density in postmenopausal Taiwanese women. Calcif Tiss Int, 60:245-9

Lau, E. M., et al., 1998. Bone mineral density in Chinese elderly female vegetarians, vegans, lacto-vegetarians and omnivores. Eur J Clin Nutr 52:60-4.

Dominguez-Rodrigo, M., et al., 2012. Earliest Porotic Hyperostosis on a 1.5-Million-Year-Old Hominin, Olduvai Gorge, Tanzania. PloS One.

Herbert, V. 1994. Staging vitamin B12 (cobalamin) in vegetarians Am J Clin Nutr 59(5):1213S-1222S.

Baker, S. J., Mollin, D. L. 1955. The Relationship between Intrinsic Factor and the Intestinal Absorption of Vitamin B12. British Journal of Haematology 1(1):46-51.

Tangney, C. C., et al., 2011. Vitamin B12, cognition, and brain MRI measures: a cross-sectional examination. Neurology 77:1276-82.

Christian, J. L., and J. L. Greger. 1994. Nutrition for Living. Red Wood City, CA: Benjaming/Cummings

Hallberg, L. 1984. Iron. In Nutrition Reviews: Present knowledge in nutrition, 5th ed, 32:459-78. Washington, D.C.: The Nutrition Foundation

Hallberg, L., et al., 1979. Dietary Heme Iron Absorption A Discussion of Possible Mechanisms for the Absorption-Promoting Effect of Meat and for the Regulation of Iron Absorption. Scandinavian Journal of Gastroenterology 14(7):769-779.

Helman, A. D., Darnton-Hill, I. 1987. Vitamin and iron status in new vegetarians. Am J Clin Nutr 45(4):785-789.

Burdge, G. C., Wooton, S. A. 2002. Conversion of alpha-linolenic acid to eicosapentaenoic, docosapentaenoic and docosahexaenoic acids in young women. Br J Nutr. 88(4):411-20.

Brenna, J. T., et al., 2009. alpha-Linolenic acid supplementation and conversion to n-3 long-chain polyunsaturated fatty acids in humans. Prostaglandins, Leukotrienes, and Essential Fatty Acids 80(2-3):85-91.

Innis, S. M. 2007. Dietary (n-3) Fatty Acids and Brain Development. J. Nutr. 137(4):855-859.

Gerster, H. 1998. Can adults adequately convert α-linolenic acid (18:3n-3) to eicosapentaenoic acid (20:5n-3) and docosahexaenoic acid (22:6n-3)? International Journal for Vitamin and Nutrition Research. 68(3):159-173.

Brouwer, I. A., Katan, M. B., Zock, P. L. 2004. Dietary α-Linolenic Acid Is Associated with Reduced Risk of Fatal Coronary Heart Disease, but Increased Prostate Cancer Risk: A Meta-Analysis. J. Nutr 134(4):919-922.

Augustsson, A., et al., 2003. Prospective Study of Intake of Fish and Marine Fatty Acids and Prostate Cancer. Cancer Epidemiol Biomarkers Prev 12; 64.

Joanne H. E. Promislow, et al., 2002. "Protein Consumption and Bone Mineral Density in the Elderly: The Rancho Bernardo Study," American Journal of Epidemiology 155, no. 7.

Cassidy CM. Eds Jerome NW et al. 1980. Nutrition and health in agriculturists and hunter-gatherers: a case study of two prehistoric populations in Nutritional Anthropology. Redgrave Publishing Company, Pleasantville, NY.

Walker, P. L., and B. S. Hewlett. Dental Health Diet and Social Status among Central African Foragers and Farmers. American Anthropologist, 92(2): 383-398.

Chavarro, J. E., Toth, T. L., Sadio, S. M., Hauser, R. 2008. Soy food and isoflavone intake in relation to semen quality parameters among men from an infertility clinic. Hum Reprod. 23(11):2584-90.

1992. Bulletin de L'Office Fédéral de la Santé Publique, no. 28.

Austringer, T. (2009, March) Effect of Soy Products on Brain Function. Retrieved From <http://www.livinghealthy360.com/index.php/effect-of-soy-products-on-brain-function-23853/>

Nagata C, Takatsuka N, Kurisu Y, Shimizu H. 1998. J Nutr 128:209-13

Circle, Sidney Joseph; Smith, Allan H. (1972). Soybeans: Chemistry and Technology. Westport, CT: Avi Publishing. pp. 104, 163.

Yildiz, Fatih (2005). Phytoestrogens in Functional Foods. Taylor & Francis Ltd. pp. 3–5, 210–211.

Turner JV, Agatonovic-Kustrin S, Glass BD. 2007. "Molecular aspects of phytoestrogen selective binding at estrogen receptors". J Pharm Sci 96 (8): 1879–1885.

Weber KS, Setchell KD, Stocco DM, Lephart ED. 2011. "Dietary soy-phytoestrogens decrease testosterone levels and prostate weight without altering LH, prostate 5alpha-reductase or testicular steroidogenic acute regulatory peptide levels in adult male Sprague-Dawley rats". J. Endocrinol. 170 (3): 591–9.

Leopold AS, Erwin M, Oh J, Browning B. 1976. "Phytoestrogens: adverse effects on reproduction in California quail". Science 191 (4222): 98–100.

De Lemos, Mário L. 2001. "Effects of Soy Phytoestrogens Genistein and Daidzein on Breast Cancer Growth". Annals of Pharmacotherapy (Harvey Whitney Books) 35 (9): 1118–1121.

Thompson LU, et al., 2006. "Phytoestrogen content of foods consumed in Canada, including isoflavones, lignans, and coumestan". Nutrition & Cancer 54(2):184–201.

Amadasi A, et al., 2008. Identification of Xenoestrogens in Food Additives by an Integrated in Silicon & in Vitro Approach. Chemical Research in Toxicology 22:52–63

Lusas, Edmund W.; Riaz, Mian N. 1995. "Soy Protein Products: Processing and Use" Journal of Nutrition (125): 573S–580S.

Blasbalg, T. L., et al., 2011. Changes in consumption of omega-3 and omega-6 fatty acids in the United States during the 20th century. Am J Clin Nutr 93(5):950-962.

Daniels, K. (2005) The Whole Soy Story: The Darkside of America's Favorite Health Food. New Trends Publishing.

Anderson, J. W., et al., 1995. "Meta-Analysis of the Effects of Soy Protein Intake on Serum Lipids". New England Journal of Medicine 333 (5): 276–282.

178

FAOSTAT. Whole soybean production in metric tonnes. Retrieved from <http://www.geohive.com/charts/ag_soybean.aspx>

Greger, J. L. 1999. Nondigestible Carbohydrates and Mineral Bioavailability. J. Nutr 129(7):1434S-1435s.

Bohn, T., et al., 2004. Phytic acid added to white-wheat bread inhibits fractional apparent magnesium absorption in humans. Am J Clin Nutr 79(3):418-423.

B E Golden, M H N Golden. 1981. Plasma zinc, rate of weight gain and the energy cost of tissue deposition in children recovering from malnutrition on cows' milk or a soya protein based diet. Am J Clin Nutr 34:892.

Committee on Food Protection, Food and Nutrition Board, National Research Council (1973). "Phytates". Toxicants Occurring Naturally in Foods. Washington, DC: National Academy of Sciences. pp. 363–371.

Yadav, S., Nhetarpaul, N. 1994. Indigenous legume fermentation: Effect on some antinutrients and in-vitro digestibility of starch and protein. Food Chemistry 50(4).

Freed, D. L. J. 1999. Do dietary lectins cause disease? BMJ 318(7190):1023-1024.

Kris-Etherton, P. M., et al., 2000. "Polyunsaturated Fatty Acids in the Food Chain in the United States," American Journal of Clinical Nutrition 71, no. 1: S179-S188

Cuatrecasas, P., Tell, G. P. E. 1973. Insulin-Like Activity of Concanavalin A and Wheat Germ Agglutinin—Direct Interactions with Insulin Receptors. Proc Natl Acad Sci U S A. 70(2): 485–489.

Nachbar, M. S., Oppenheim, J. D. 1980. Lectins in the United States diet: a survey of lectins in commonly consumed foods and a review of the literature. Am J Clin Nutr 33(11):2338-2345.

Micha, R., Wallace, S. K., Mozaffarian, D. 2010. Red and processed meat consumption and risk of incident coronary heart disease, stroke, and diabetes mellitus: a systematic review and meta-analysis. Circulation 121(21):2271-83.

Rohrmann, S., et al., 2013. Meat consumption and mortality--results from the European Prospective Investigation into Cancer and Nutrition. BMC Med. 11:63.

Alexander, D. D., et al., 2011. Meta-analysis of prospective studies of red meat consumption and colorectal cancer. Eur J Cancer Prev. 20(4):293-307.

Alexander, D. D., Cushing, C. A. 2011. Red meat and colorectal cancer: a critical summary of prospective epidemiologic studies. Obes Rev. 12(5):e472-93.

Wynder, E. L., et al., 1975. J Natl Can Inst 54:7.

179

MG Enig. (2000) Know Your Fats: The Complete Primer for Understanding the Nutrition of Fats, Oils, and Cholesterol. (Bethesda Press; MD.), 84-85.

M Gaard et al., 1996. Dietary factors and risk of colon cancer: a prospective study of 50,535 young Norwegian men and women. Eur J Cancer Prev, 5:445-54.

de Stefani, E., et al., 1997. Meat intake, heterocyclic amines, and risk of breast cancer: a case-control study in Uruguay. Cancer Epidemiol Biom Prev, 6:573-81

Abrams, H. L. 2000. Vegetarianism: another view, in The Cambridge World History of Food. K Kiple and K Ornelas, editors. (Cambridge University Press; UK), 2(1567).

Dwyer, J. 1979. Vegetarianism. Contemporary Nutr, 4:1-2.

Lyon, J. L., et al., 1976. Cancer incidence in Mormons and non-Mormons in Utah, 1966-1970. New Eng J Med, 294:129.

Mills, J., et al., 1994. Cancer-incidence among California Seventh-day Adventists, 1976-1982. Am J Clin Nutr 59 (suppl):1136S-42S;

Phillips, R. L., 1975. Role of life-style and dietary habits in risk of cancer among Seventh Day AdventistsCanc Res 35:3513-3522

Lehrke, S., et al., 2009. Prediction of coronary artery disease by a systemic atherosclerosis score index derived from whole-body MR angiography. J Cardiovasc Magn Reson 11(1):36.

Burr, M. L., Sweetnam, P. M. 1992. Vegetarianism, dietary fiber, and mortality. Am J Clin Nutr 36(5):873-7.

Roosevelt, F. D. 1937. Letter to all state governors on a uniform soil conservation law. The American Presidency Project.

Smith, R., and E Pinckney. 1998. Diet, Blood Cholesterol, and Coronary Heart Disease: A Critical Review of the Literature--vol. 2. (Vector Enterprises; CA). Jnl of PPNF 22:4: 27-29.

Burr, M. L., and PM Sweetnam. 1982. Vegetarianism, dietary fiber, and mortality. Amer J Clin Nutr, 36:873.

Abrams, H. L. 1979. The relevance of paleolithic diet in determining contemporary nutritional needs. J Appl Nutr 31:1,2:43-59.

Mistake #3

Cordain, L., et al., 2000. Plant-animal subsistence ratios and macronutrient energy estimations in worldwide hunter-gatherer diets. Am J Clin Nutr 71(3):682-692.

DJ Stanford and JA Day, (1992) Ice Age Hunters of the Rockies. (University Press of Colorado; CO.)

Fallon, S., and MG Enig. Caveman Cuisine. Jnl of PPNF, 21:2:1-4.

Cordain, L. The Paleo Diet. 2010. Houghton Mifflin Harcourt.

Richards, M. P. 2002. A brief review of the archaeological evidence for Paleolithic and Neolithic subsistence. European Journal of Clinical Nutrition 56

Boyd Eaton S., and M. Konner. 1985. cited in the New England Journal of Medicine ("Paleolithic nutrition: a consideration of its nature and current implications." N. Eng. J. Med. 321:283–289.

Wolf, R.(2010) The Paleo Solution: The Original Human Diet. Las Vegas: Victory Bell

Keys A. 1953. "Atherosclerosis: a problem in newer public health". Journal of the Mount Sinai Hospital, New York 20 (2): 118–39.

Marmot, M.G. 1985. Interpretation of Trends in Coronary Heart Disease Mortality. Acta Med Scand 701: 58.

Artaud-Wild SM, et al., 1993. Differences in coronary mortality can be explained by differences in cholesterol and saturated fat intakes in 40 countries but not in France and Finland. A paradox. Circulation 88:2771–9

Siri-Tarino, P. W., et al., 2010. Meta-analysis of prospective cohort studies evaluating the association of saturated fat with cardiovascular disease. Am J Clin Nutr 27725.

Erickson, K. L. 1984. Dietary fat influences on murine melanoma growth and lymphocyte-mediated cytotoxicity. J Natl Cancer Inst. 72(1):115-20.

Centers for Disease Control and Prevention. 2004. Trends in intake of energy and macronutrients--United States, 1971-2000. MMWR Morb Mortal Wkly Rep. 53(4):80-2.

Enig, M. 1995. Trans Fatty Acids in the Food Supply: A Comprehensive Report Covering 60 Years of Research, 2nd edition. (Enig Associates; MD)

Mistake #4

Perlmutter, D., and Kristin Loberg. 2013. Grain Brain: The Surprising Truth About Wheat, Carbs, and Sugar – Your Brain's Silent Killers. New York: Little, Brown and Company. Pg. 187-188.

Virchow, Rudolf. 1856. "Gesammelte Abhandlungen zur wissenschaftlichen Medizin". Vierteljahrschrift für die praktische Heilkunde (Germany: Staatsdruckerei Frankfurt). Phlogose und Thrombose im Gefäßsystem.

Anitschkow NN, Chatalov S. 1913. "Über experimentelle Cholesterinsteatose und ihre Bedeutung für die Entstehung einiger pathologischer Prozesse". Zentralbl Allg Pathol 24: 1–9.

Anitschkow NN. 1913. "Über die Veränderungen der Kaninchenaorta bei experimenteller Cholesterinsteatose". Beitr Pathol Anat 56: 379–404.

Duff GL, McMillian GC. 1951. "Pathology of atherosclerosis". Am J Med 11 (1): 92–108

Norum KR. 1978. "Some present concepts concerning diet and prevention of coronary heart disease.". Nutr Metab 22 (1): 1–7.

NIH Consensus Development Conference, JAMA 1985, 253:2080

Steinberg D 2006. "Thematic review series: the pathogenesis of atherosclerosis. An interpretive history of the cholesterol controversy, part V: the discovery of the statins and the end of the controversy". J. Lipid Res. 47 (7):1339–51.

Ravnskov, Uffe (2000). The Cholesterol Myths: Exposing the Fallacy that Saturated Fat and Cholesterol cause Heart Disease. United States: New Trends Publishing.

Ravnskov Uffe (1992). "Cholesterol lowering trials in coronary heart disease: frequency of citation and outcome". British Medical Journal 305 (6844): 15–19, 420–422, 717.

Ravnskov U. 1995. "Quotation bias in reviews of the diet-heart idea", Journal of Clinical Epidemiology 48: 713-9.

Ravnskov U. 2002. "Debatt i Science: Kostråd mot hjärtinfarkt försvaras med felcitat", Läkartidningen 99: 2673.

Ravnskov U., et al., 2002. "Studies of dietary fat and heart disease", Science 295: 1464-5.

Rifkind B, Levy R. 1978. "Testing the lipid hypothesis. Clinical trials". Archives of surgery (Chicago, Ill. : 1960) 113 (1): 80–3.

Oliver M. 1981. "Lipid lowering and ischaemic heart disease". Acta Med. Scand. Suppl. 651: 285–93.

Stehbens W (1988). "Flaws in the lipid hypothesis of atherogenesis". Pathology 20 (4): 395–6.

de Lorgeril, M. et al., 1999. "Mediterranean Diet, Traditional Risk Factors, and the Rate of Cardiovascular Complications After Myocardial Infarction: Final Report of the Lyon Diet Heart Study," Circulation 99:779-785

Braumwald, E. 1997. "Shattuck Lecture: Cardiovascular Medicine at the Turn of the Millennium: Triumphs, Concerns, and Opportunities," New England Journal of Medicine 337(19):1360-1369.

Prior, I., et al., 1981. "Cholesterol, Coconuts, and Diet on Polynesian Atolls: A Natural Experiment: The Pukapuka and Tokelau Island Studies," American Journal of Clinical Nutrition 34(8):1552-1561.

Krumholz, H. M., et al., 1994. "Lack of Association between Cholesterol and Coronary Heart Disease Mortality and Morbidity and All-Case Mortality In Persons Older than 70 Years," Journal of the American Medical Association 272(17):1335-1340.

McMurray, W. 1977. Essentials of Human Metabolism. New York: Harper & Row.

Stehbens WE. 2001. "Coronary heart disease, hypercholesterolemia, and atherosclerosis I. False premises". Exp Mol Pathol 70 (2): 103–119.

Mann GV. 1977. Diet-heart: end of an era. New England Journal of Medicine 297:644-650.

Kannel, W. B., and T Gordon. 1970. The Framingham Diet Study: diet and the regulations of serum cholesterol (Sect 24). Washington DC, Dept of Health, Education and Welfare.

Superko HR, Nejedly M, Garrett B. 2002. Small LDL and its clinical importance as a new CAD risk factor: a female case study. Prog Cardiovasc Nurs 17:167–73.

Nichols, A. B., et al. 1976. Daily nutritional intake and serum lipid levels: The Tecumseh Study. Am J Clin Nutr . 29: 1384.

1982. Multiple Risk Factor Intervention Trial. JAMA . 248: 1465.

Elias, P. K., et al., 2005. "Serum Cholesterol and Cognitive Performance in the Framingham Heart Study," Psychosomatic Medicine 67(1):24-30.

West, R., et al., 2008. "Better Memory Functioning Associated with Higher Total and Low-density Lipoprotein Cholesterol Levels in Very Elderly Subjects Without and Apolipoprotein e4 Allele." American Journal of Geriatric Psychiatry 16(9):781:85.

Dawber, T. R. 1980. The Framingham Study. Cambridge, M.A.: Harvard University Press.

183

Powell, K. E. et al. 1987. Physical activity and the incidence of coronary artery disease. Annual Review of Public Health 8:253-87.

Brown, D. R. 1990. Exercise, fitness, and mental health. In Exercise, Fitness, and Health, ed. 607-26. Champaign, IL: Human Kinetics.

Reaven, G. M. 1988. Role of insulin resistance in human disease. Diabetes 37:1595-1607.

Kannel, W. B. 1990. Contribution of the Framingham Study to prevent cardiovascular disease. Journal of the American College of Cardiology 15:206-11.

Paffenbarger, R. S., et al., 1986. Physical activity, all cause mortality, and longevity of college alumni. New England Journal of Medicine 315 (March 6):605-13.

Jacobs, D., et al., 1992. "Report of the Conference on Low Blood Cholesterol: Mortality Associations," Circulation 86, no. 3:1046-60.

Huang, X., et al., 2008. "Low LDL Cholesterol and Increased Risk of Parkinson's Disease: Prospective Results from Honolulu-Asia Aging Study." Movement Disorders 23, no.7:1013-18.

De Lau, L. M., et al., 2006. "Serum Cholesterol Levels and the Risk of Parkinson's Disease." American Journal of Epidemiology 164, no. 10:998-1002.

Shin, J. Y., et al., 2008. "Are Cholesterol and Depression Inversely Related? A Meta-analysis of the Association Between Two Cardiac Risk Factors." Annals of Behavioral Medicine 36(1):33-43.

Morgan, R. E., et al., 1993. "Plasma Cholesterol and Depressive Symptoms in Older Men." Lancet 341(8837):75-79.

Horsten, M. et al., 1997. "Depressive Symptoms, Social Support, and Lipid Profile in Healthy Middle-aged Women." Psychosomatic Medicine 59(5):521-28.

Steegmans, P. H., et al., 2000. "Higher Prevalence of Depressive Symptoms in Middle-aged Men with Low Serum Cholesterol Levels." Psychosomatic Medicine 62(2):205-11.

Perez-Rodriguez, M. M., et al., 2008. "Low Serum Cholesterol May Be Associated with Suicide Attempt History." Journal of Clinical Psychiatry 69(12):1920-27.

Boscarino, J. A., et al., 2009. "Low Serum Cholesterol and External-cause Mortality: Potential Implications for Research and Surveillance." Journal of Psychiatric Research 43(9):848-54.

Travison, T. G., et al., 2007. A Population-Level Decline in Serum Testosterone Levels in American Men. The Journal of Clinical Endocrinology & Metabolism. 92(1).

Rizvi, K., et al., 2002. "Do Lipid-Lowering Drugs Cause Erectile Dysfunction? A Systematic Review." Journal of the Family Practice 19, no. 1:95-98.

Corona, G., et al., 2010. "The Effect of Statin Therapy on Testosterone Levels in Subjects Consulting for Erectile Dysfunction." Journal of Sexual Medicine 7, no. 4:1547-56.

Golomb, B. A., Evans, M. A. 2008. Statin adverse effects : a review of the literature and evidence for a mitochondrial mechanism. Am J Cardiovasc Drugs. 8(6):373-418.

Charach, G., et al., 2010. "Baseline Low-density Lipoprotein Cholesterol Levels and Outcome in Patients with Heart Failure." American Journal of Cardiology 105, no. 1:100-04.

Seneff, S., "APOE-4: The Clue to Why Low Fat Diet and Statins May Cause Alzheimer's" (December 2009), http://people.csail.mit.edu/seneff/alzheimers_statins.html

Taubes G (March 2001). "Nutrition. The soft science of dietary fat". Science 291 (5513): 2536–45.

Gaziano, J. M. 1997. "Fasting Triglycerides, High-Density Lipoprotein, and Risk of Myocardial Infarction," Circulation 96:2520-2525.

Nelson GJ, Schmidt PC, Kelley DS. 1995. Low-fat diets do not lower plasma cholesterol levels in healthy men compared to high-fat diets with similar fatty acid composition at constant caloric intake. Lipids. 30:969-976

Mistake #5

Ramsden, C. (2013, February) Study raises questions about dietary fats and heart disease guidance. British Medical Journal. Retrieved from < http://www.bmj.com/press-releases/2013/02/04/study-raises-questions-about-dietary-fats-and-heart-disease-guidance>

Dreon, D. M., et al., Reduced LDL particle size in children consuming a very-low-fat diet is related to parental LDL-subclass patterns. Am J Clin Nutr June 71(6):1611-1616.

Dreon, D. M., et al., 1999. A very low-fat diet is not associated with improved lipoprotein profiles in men with a predominance of large, low-density lipoproteins. Am J Clin Nutr. 69(3):411-8.

Brinton, E. A., et al., 1990. A low-fat diet decreases high density lipoprotein (HDL) cholesterol levels by decreasing HDL apolipoprotein transport rates. J Clin Invest. 85(1):144–151.

Asztalos, B., et al., Differential response to low-fat diet between low and normal HDL-cholesterol subjects. The Journal of Lipid Research 41:321-328.

Katan, M. B. 1998. Effect of low-fat diets on plasma high-density lipoprotein concentrations. Am J Clin Nutr. 67(3 Suppl):573S-576S.

M G Marmot. 1985. Interpretation of Trends in Coronary Heart Disease Mortality. Acta Med Scand 701: 58.

Willett, W. C., et al. 1993. Intake of trans fatty acids and risk of coronary heart disease among women. Lancet 341: 581.

Aiello LC, Wheeler P. 1995. The expensive-tissue hypothesis: The brain and the digestive system in human and primate evolution. Current Anthropology 36(2): 199–221.

Nenseter MS, Drevon CA. 1996. Dietary polyunsaturates and peroxidation of low density lipoprotein. Curr Opin Lipidol. 7(1):8-13.
Jenkinson, A., et al., 1999. Dietary intakes of polyunsaturated fatty acids and indices of oxidative stress in human volunteers. European Journal of Clinical Nutrition 53(7):523-528.

Harman D. 2009. Origin and evolution of the free radical theory of aging: a brief personal history, 1954–2009. Biogerontology. 10(6) 773-81.

Clancy D, Birdsall J. Flies, worms and the Free Radical Theory of ageing. Ageing Research Reviews

Dizdaroglu M, Jaruga P. 2012. Mechanisms of free radical-induced damage to DNA. Free Radical Research. 46(4) 382-419.

Draper HH, McGirr LG, Hadley M. 1986. The metabolism of malondialdehyde. Lipids 21: 305–307.

Halliwell B, Chirico S. 1993. Lipid peroxidation: its mechanism, measurement, significance. Am J Clin Nutr 57: 715S–725S.

Calder, P. C. 2006. n–3 Polyunsaturated fatty acids, inflammation, and inflammatory diseases. Am J Clin Nutr 83(6):S1505-1519S

Simopoulos, A.P. 2002. "The importance of the ratio of omega-6/omega-3 essential fatty acids". Biomedicine & Pharmacotherapy 56 (8): 365–79.

Holub, B. J., et al., 2009. Correlation of omega-3 levels in serum phospholipid from 2053 human blood samples with key fatty acid ratios. Nutrition Journal 8:58.

Ramsden, C. E., et al., 2010. n-6 fatty acid-specific and mixed polyunsaturate dietary interventions have different effects on CHD risk: a meta-analysis of randomised controlled trials. Br J Nutr. 104(11):1586-600.

Christakis, M. D., et al., 1966. Effect of the Anti-Coronary Club Program on Coronary Heart Disease Risk-Factor Status. JAMA. 198(6):597-604.

Kris-Etherton, P. M., et al., 2000. "Polyunsaturated Fatty Acids in the Food Chain in the United States," American Journal of Clinical Nutrition 71, no. 1: S179-S188;

Sonestedt, E., et al., 2008. "Do Both Heterocyclic Amines and Omega-6 Polyunsaturated Fatty Acids Contribute to the Incidence of Breast Cancer in Postmenopausal Women of the Malmö Diet and Cancer Cohort?". International Journal of Cancer (John Wiley & Sons) 123 (7): 1637–1643.

Dantzer R, et al., 2008. From inflammation to sickness and depression: when the immune system subjugates the brain. Nat Rev Neurosci. 9(1):46-56

Lenoard BE. 2007. Inflammation, depression, and dementia: are they connected? Neurochem Res. 2007 Oct;32(10):1749-56.

M. A. French, K. Sundram, and M.T. Clandinin. 2002. "Cholesterolaemic Effect of Palmitic Acid in Relation to Other Dietary Fatty Acids," Asia Pacific Journal of Clinical Nutrition 11 (7): S401-S407.

Ascherio, A., Willet, W. C. Health effects of trans fatty acids. Am J Clin Nutr 66(4): 1006S-1010S.

Mensink, R. P., Katan, M. B. 1990. Effect of Dietary trans Fatty Acids on High-Density and Low-Density Lipoprotein Cholesterol Levels in Healthy Subjects. N Engl J Med 323:439-445.

Lopez-Garcia, E., et al., 2005. Consumption of Trans Fatty Acids Is Related to Plasma Biomarkers of Inflammation and Endothelial Dysfunction. J. Nutr. 135(3):562-566

Lichtenstein, A. H. 1997. Trans Fatty Acids, Plasma Lipid Levels, and Risk of Developing Cardiovascular Disease: A Statement for Healthcare Professionals From the American Heart Association. Circulation 95:2588-2590

Gillman MW, et al. 1997. Margarine intake and subsequent coronary heart disease in men. Epidemiology

Mary G. Enig, (2000) Know Your Fats: The Complete Primer for Understanding the Nutrition of Fats, Oils, and Cholesterol. Brookhaven, PA: Bethesda Press.

Willet, W. C., and Ascherio, A. 1994. "Commentary: Trans-Fatty Acids: Are the Effects Only Marginal?" American Journal of Public Health 84:722-724

Mann, B. V. 1994. "Metabolic Consequences of Dietary Trans-Fatty Acids," Lancet 343:1268-1271.

Salmeron, J. et al., 2001. Dietary Fat Intake and Risk of Type 2 Diabetes in Women," American Journal of Clinical Nutrition 73, no. 6:1019-1026

Micha, R., Mozaffarian, D. 2008. Trans Fatty Acids: Effect on Cardiometabolic Health and Implications for Policy. Prostaglandins, Leukotrienes, and Essential Fatty Acids. 79(3-5), 147-152.

Ruano, c., et al. 2011. Dietary Fat intake and Quality of Life: The Sun Project. Nutrition Journal. 10, 121.

Golomb, B., Evans, M., et al. Trans-Fat Consumption and Aggression. PLoS One. 201. 7(3), 32175.

Wolk, A. et al. 1998. A Prospective Study of Association of Monounsaturated Fat and Other Types of Fat With Risk of Breast Cancer. Arch Intern Med .158: 41-45

Balter, M. 1991. Europe: as many cancers as cuisines. Science 254: 114

Koh, H. K. 1991. Cutaneous melanoma. N Eng J Med 325: 171.

Kearney, R. 1987. Promotion and prevention of tumour growth -effects of endotoxin, inflammation and dietary lipids. Int Clin Nutr Rev 7: 157.

Ip, C., Scimeca, J. A., Thompson H. 1995. Effect of timing and duration of dietary conjugated linoleic acid on mammary cancer prevention. Nutr Cancer. 24: 241.

Mistake #6

Institute of Medicine (IOM) of the National Academies, "Dietary Reference Intakes, Energy, Carbohydrate, Fiber, Fat, Fatty Acids, Cholesterol, Protein, and Amino Acids." Washington, DC: National Academies Press (2002), pg. 275.

Harper AE. 1999. Defining the essentiality of nutrients. In: Shils MD, Olson JA, Shihe M, Ross AC, eds. Modern nutrition in health and disease. 9th ed. Boston: William and Wilkins, 3–10.

Manninen, A. H. 2004. "Metabolic Effects of the Very-Low Carbohydrate Diets: Misunderstood 'Villains' of Human Metabolism," Journal of the International Society of Sports Nutrition 1, no.2:7-11.

Manninen, A. H. 2006. Very-low carbohydrate diets and preservation of muscle mass. Nutr Metab (Lond). 3:9.

Cahill GF. 1970. Starvation in man. N Engl J Med 282:668–75.

Phinney, S. D. 2004. Ketogenic diets and physical performance. Nutrition & Metabolism 1:2.

Kaye-Foster Powell, Susanna H. A. Holt, Janette C. Brand-Miller. 2002. "International Table of Glycemic Index and Glycemic Load Values," American Journal of Clinical Nutrition 76, no. 1:5-56.

Ebert, D; Haller, RG; Walton, ME. 2003. "Energy contribution of octanoate to intact rat brain metabolism measured by 13C nuclear magnetic resonance spectroscopy.". The Journal of neuroscience : the official journal of the Society for Neuroscience 23 (13): 5928–35.

Hultman, E. 1967. Physiological role of muscle glycogen in man with special reference to exercise. In Circulation Research XX and XX1, ed. C. B. Chapman, 1-99 and 1-114, New York: The American Heart Association.

Raatz SK, Bibus D, Thomas W, Kris-Etherton P. 2001. Total fat intake modifies plasma fatty acid composition in humans. J Nutr. 131(2):231-4.

King IB, Lemaitre RN, Kestin M. 2006. Effect of a low-fat diet on fatty acid composition in red cells, plasma phospholipids, and cholesterol esters: investigation of a biomarker of total fat intake. Am J Clin Nutr. 83(2):227-36.

Young CM, Scanlan SS, Im HS, Lutwak L. 1971. Effect of body composi-tion and other parameters in obese young men of carbohy-drate level of reduction diet. Am J Clin Nutr 24:290-6

Bellisari, A. 2008. Evolutionary origins of obesity. Bellisari A. Obes Rev. 9(2):165-80.

Eaton, S. B., et al., 2009. Evolution, body composition, insulin receptor competition, and insulin resistance. Prev Med. 49:283-85

Laycock, J. F., and P. H. Wise. 1983. Essential Endocrinology. New York: Oxford University Press.

Kopp, W. 2003. High-insulinogenic nutrition-an etiologic factor for obesity and the metabolic syndrome? Kopp W. Metabolism. 52(7):840-4.

Sanchez-Lozada, L. G., et al., 2008. How safe is fructose for persons with or without diabetes? Sanchez-Lozada LG, Le M, Segal M, Johnson RJ. Am J Clin Nutr. 88(5):1189-90.

189

Sonksen, P., Sonksen, P., 2000. Insulin: understanding its action in health and disease. Br J Anaesth. 85(1):69-79.

Unger RH, Scherer PH. 2010. Gluttony, sloth and the metabolic syndrome: a roadmap to lipotoxicity. Trends Endocrinal Metab. 21(6):345-52. Epub 2010 Mar 10.

Appleton, N. (1996). Lick the Sugar Habit (New York: Avery)

Stocker, R., and Keaney Jr., J. F., 2004. "Role of Oxidative Modifications in Atherosclerosis," Physiology Review 84, no. 4:1381-1478.

Seyfried TN, Shelton LM. 2010. Cancer as a metabolic disease. Nutr Metab (Lond). 27;7:7.

Giovannucci E. 2003. Nutrition, insulin, insulin-like growth factors and cancer. Horm Metab Res. 35(11-12):694-704.

Cordain L. Medikament. 2001. Syndrome X: Just the tip of the hyperinsulinemia iceberg. 6:46-51

Cordain L, Eades MR, Eades MD. 2003. Hyperinsulinemic disease of civilization: more than just Syndrom X. Comp Biochem Physiol A Mol Integr Physiol. 136(1):95-112.

Ausk KJ, Boyko EJ, Ioannou GN. 2010. Insulin resistance predicted mortality in nondiabetic individuals in the U.S. Diabetes Care. 33(6):1179-85.

Francheschi S. et al., 1996. Intake of macronutrients and risk of breast cancer. Lancet 347:1351-6

Lutz, W. J. 1995. The colonization of Europe and our Western diseases. Med Hypotheses, 45:115-120.

Witte, J. et al., 1997. Diet and premenopausal bilateral breast cancer: a case control study. Breast Canc Res & Treat, 42:243-251;

Francheschi, S. et al., 1997. Food groups and risk of colo-rectal cancer in Italy. Inter J Canc, 72:56-61

Seely, S. et al., 1985. Diet Related Diseases--The Modern Epidemic (AVI Publishing; CT), 190-200.

Stefansson, V. Cancer: Disease of Civilization. (Hill and Wang; NY), 1960.

Bidoli, E., R. et al., 2005. Macronutrients, fatty acids, cholesterol, and prostate cancer. Annals of Oncology 16: 152-157

190

Edefonti, V., Decarli, A., La Vecchia, C., Bosetti, C., Randi, G., Franceschi, S. Dal Maso, L., Ferraroni, M. 2008. Nutrient dietary patterns and the risk of breast and ovarian cancers. International Journal of Cancer 122(3): 609-13

Fall, T., et al., 2013. The Role of Adiposity in Cardiometabolic Traits: A Mendelian Randomization Analysis. PLoS Medicine, 10 (6): e1001474

Mistake #7

Khaw, K. T., et al., 1987. Dietary fiber and reduced ischemic heart disease mortality rates in men and women: a 12-year prospective study. Am J Epidemiol. 126(6):1093-102.

Ma, Y., et al., 2008. Association between dietary fiber and markers of systemic inflammation in the Women's Health Initiative Observational Study. Nutrition. 24(10):941-9.

Wu, H., et al., 2003. Dietary fiber and progression of atherosclerosis: the Los Angeles Atherosclerosis Study. Am J Clin Nutr 78(6):1085-1091.

Aune, D., et al., 2011. Dietary fibre, whole grains, and risk of colorectal cancer: systematic review and dose-response meta-analysis of prospective studies. BMJ 343

Whorton, J. 2000. Civilization and the colon: constipation as the "disease of diseases." British Medical Journal 321(7276):1586-89.

Burkitt, D. P., et al. 1963. Some geographical variations in disease patterns in East and Central Africa. E Afr Med J . 40: 1.

Burkitt D. P. 1979. Epidemiology of cancer of the colon and rectum. Cancer 28:3-13.

Mann, G. V. et al., 1972. "Atherosclerosis in the Masai," American Journal of Epidemiology 95:26-37.

Lyon, J. L., et al., 1976. Cancer incidence in Mormons and non-Mormons in Utah, 1966-1970. New Eng J Med, 294:129.

1973. Dietary fiber, ischaemic heart disease and diabetes mellitus. Proc Nutr Soc. 32: 151.

Swain, J. F., et al., 1990. Comparison of the Effects of Oat Bran and Low-Fiber Wheat on Serum Lipoprotein Levels and Blood Pressure. N Engl J Med 322:147-152

Brown, L., et al., 1999. Cholesterol-lowering effects of dietary fiber: a meta-analysis. Am J Clin Nutr. 69(1):30-42.

Burr, M. L., et al., 1989. Diet and reinfarction trial (DART): design, recruitment, and compliance. Eur Heart J. 1989 10(6):558-67.

Mcintosh, M. et al., 2001. A Diet Containing Food Rich in Soluble and Insoluble Fiber Improves Glycemic Control and Reduces Hyperlipidemia Among Patients with Type 2 Diabetes Mellitus. Nutrition Reviews 59(2):52-55.

Harland, B. F. 1989. Dietary fibre and mineral bioavailability. Nutr Res Rev. 2(1):133-47.

Norman, D., et al. 1987. The impact of dietary fat and fiber on intestinal carcinogenesis. Prev Med. (4): 554.

Harland, B. F. 1989. Dietary fibre and mineral bioavailability. Nutr Res Rev. 2(1):133-47.

Boyd Eaton, S. and M. Konner, 1985. "Paleolithic nutrition: a consideration of its nature and current implications." N. Eng. J. Med. 321, 283–289

Lindeberg, S. et al. 2007. A Palaeolithic diet improves glucose tolerance more than a Mediterranean-like diet in individuals with ischaemic heart disease. Diabetologia 50, 1795-1807.

Braly, J. with Hoggan, R. (2002) Dangerous Grains (New York: Avery)

Williams, P. 2011. Evaluation of the Evidence Between Consumption of Refined Grains and Health Outcomes. Nutrition Reviews. 70(2), 80-99.

Spreadbury, I., et al. 2012. Comparison with Ancestral Diets Suggests Dense Acellular Carbohydrates Promote Inflammatory Microbiota, and May Be The Primary Dietary Cause of Leptin Resistance and Obesity. Diabetes, Metabolic Syndrome, and Obesity: Targets and Therapy. 5, 175-189.

Lindgarde F, Widen I, Gebb M, Ahren B. 2004. Traditional versus agricultural lifestyle among Shuar women of the Ecuadorian Amazon: effects on leptin levels. Metabolism. 53(10):1355–1358.

Page LB, Damon A, Moellering RC., Jr. 1974. Antecedents of cardiovascular disease in six Solomon Islands societies. Circulation. 49(6):1132–1146.

de La Serre CB, Ellis CL, Lee J, Hartman AL, Rutledge JC, Raybould HE. 2010. Propensity to high-fat diet-induced obesity in rats is associated with changes in the gut microbiota and gut inflammation. Am J Physiol Gastrointest Liver Physiol. 299(2):G440–G448.

Ding S, Chi MM, Scull BP, et al. 2010. High-fat diet: bacteria interactions promote intestinal inflammation which precedes and correlates with obesity and insulin resistance in mouse. PLoS One. 5(8):e12191

Lumeng CN, Saltiel AR. 2011. Inflammatory links between obesity and metabolic disease. J Clin Invest. 121(6):2111–2117.

Lassenius MI, Pietilainen KH, Kaartinen K, et al. 2011. Bacterial endotoxin activity in human serum is associated with dyslipidemia, insulin resistance, obesity, and chronic inflammation. Diabetes Care. 34(8):1809–1815.

Ghanim H, Abuaysheh S, Sia CL, et al. 2009. Increase in plasma endotoxin concentrations and the expression of Toll-like receptors and suppressor of cytokine signaling-3 in mononuclear cells after a high-fat, high-carbohydrate meal: implications for insulin resistance. Diabetes Care. 32(12):2281–2287.

Caesar R, Reigstad CS, Backhed HK, et al. 2012. Gut-derived lipopolysaccharide augments adipose macrophage accumulation but is not essential for impaired glucose or insulin tolerance in mice. Gut

Miyake K, Tanaka T, McNeil PL. 2007. "Lectin-Based Food Poisoning: A New Mechanism of Protein Toxicity". In Steinhardt, Richard. PLoS ONE 2 (1): e687.

Jonsson T, Olsson S, Ahren B, Bog-Hansen TC, Dole A, Lindeberg S. 2005. Agrarian diet and diseases of affluence – do evolutionary novel dietary lectins cause leptin resistance? BMC Endocr Disord. 5:10.

Harris, L. A. 2005. Chronic constipation: Mechanisms of action and effective treatment. Advanced Studies in Medicine 6(10b).

Brandt, L. J., et al., 2002. Systematic review on the management of irritable bowel syndrome in North America. Am J Gastroenterol. 97(11 Suppl):S7-26.

C Y Francis, P J Whorwell. 1994. Bran and irritable bowel syndrome: time for reappraisal. Lancet 344: 39.

Hallberg, L. 1987. Wheat fiber, phytates and iron absorption. Scand J Gastroenterol Suppl. 129:73-9.

Hallberg, L., et al. 1987. Phytates and the inhibitory effect of bran on iron absorption in man. Am J Clin Nutr. 45(5): 988

Kelsay, J. L., et al., 1979. Effect of fiber from fruits and vegetables on metabolic responses of human subjects, II. Calcium, magnesium, iron, and silicon balances. Am J Clin Nutr. 32(9):1876-80.

Navert, B., et al., 1985. Reduction of the phytate content of bran by leavening in bread and its effect on zinc absorption in man. Br J Nutr. 53(1):47-53.

Gerutti, G., et al. Phytic acid in bran and in 'natural' foods. Bolletino Chimico Farmaceutico, Milan.

Stevens, J., et al. 1987. Effect of psyllium gum and wheat bran on spontaneous energy intake. Am J Clin Nutr. 46: 812.

Turnlund, J. R., et al. 1984. A stable isotope study of zinc absorption in young men: effects of phytate and alpha-cellulose. Am J Clin Nutr. 40: 1071.

Hallberg, L., et al. 1987. Phytates and the inhibitory effect of bran on iron absorption in man. Am J Clin Nutr. 45(5): 988.

Balasubraminian, R., et al. 1987. Effect of wheat bran on bowel function and fecal calcium in older adults. J Am Coll Nutr . 6(3): 199.

Bohn, T., et al., 2004. Phytic acid added to white-wheat bread inhibits fractional apparent magnesium absorption in humans. Am J Clin Nutr. 79(3):418-23.

Hughes, R. E., Johns, E. 1985. Apparent relation between dietary fiber and reproductive function in the female. Ann Hum Biol. 12: 325.;

Lloyd, T. et al. 1987. Inter-relationships of diet, athletic activity, menstrual status and bone density in collegiate women. Am J Clin Nutr. 46: 681.

Southgate, D. A. T. 1987. Minerals, trace elements and potential hazards. Am J Clin Nutr. 45:1256.

Anderson, J., et al, 2012. Health Benefits of Dietary Fiber. Nutrition Reviews. 67(4), 188-205.

Seow, A., et al., 2006. Diabetes Mellitus and Risk of Colorectal Cancer in the Singapore Chinese Health Study. JNCI J Natl Cancer Inst 98(2):135-138.

Aune, D., et al., 2011. Dietary fibre, whole grains, and risk of colorectal cancer: systematic review and dose-response meta-analysis of prospective studies. BMJ 343

Mistake #8

Schwartz, B. (2004) The Paradox of Choice: Why More is Less – How the Culture of Abundance Robs us of Satisfaction. (New York: Harper Collins) ch. 3, pg. 61.

O'Keefe JH, Cordain L. 2004. Cardiovascular disease resulting from a diet and lifestyle at odds with our Paleolithic genome: How to become a 21st-century hunter-gatherer. Mayo Clin Proc 79:101-108

St Jeor ST, Howard BV, Prewitt E, et al.. 2001. Dietary protein and weight reduction: A statement for health care professionals from the Nutrition Committee of the Council on Nutrition, Physical Activity, and Metabolism of the American Heart Association. Circulation104:1869-1874.

194

Manninen, A. H. 2004. High-Protein Weight Loss Diets and Purported Adverse Effects: Where is the Evidence? Journal of the International Society of Sports Nutrition 1:45-51.

Knight, E. L. et al., 2003. "The Impact of Protein Intake on Renal Function Decline in Women with Normal Renal Function or Mild Renal Insufficiency," Annals of Internal Medicine 138:460-467.

Rosenvinge Skov, A. et al., 1999. "Changes in Renal Function During Weight Loss Induced by High vs. Low-Protein Low-Fat Diets in Overweight Subjects," International Journal of Obesity and Related Metabolic Disorders 23(11):1170-1177.

Martin, W. F., 2005. Dietary protein intake and renal function. Nutrition & Metabolism 2:25.

Wiegmann, T. B., et al., 1990. "Controlled Changes in Chronic Dietary Protein Intake Do No Change Glomerular Filtration Rate," American Journal of Kidney Disease, no. 2:147-154.

Friedman, A. N., et al., Comparative Effects of Low-Carbohydrate High-Protein Versus Low-Fat Diets on the Kidney. CJASN 7(7): 1103-1111.

Martin, W. F., 2005. Dietary protein intake and renal function. Nutrition & Metabolism 2:25.

Poortmans, J. R., Dellalieux, O. 2000. Do regular high protein diets have potential health risks on kidney function in athletes? International Journal of Sports Nutrition 10(1):28-38.

Walser M. 1999. Effects of protein intake on renal function and on the development of renal disease. In The Role of Protein and Amino Acids in Sustaining and Enhancing Performance. Committee on Military Nutrition Research, Institute of Medicine. Washington, DC: National Academies Press 137-154.

Klahr S, Levey AS, Beck GJ, et al. 1994. The effects of dietary protein restriction and blood-pressure control on the progression of chronic renal failure. N Engl J Med 330:877-884.

Ikizler TA. 2003. Nutrition support and management of renal disorders. In Nutritional Aspects and Clinical Management of Chronic Disorders and Diseases. Edited by Bronner F. Boca Raton, FL: CRC Press 156-175.

Gougeon-Reyburn, R., et al., 1989. Comparison of daily diets containing 400 kcal (1.67 MJ) of either protein or glucose, and their effects on the response to subsequent total fasting in obese subjects. Am J Clin Nutr. 50(4):746-58.

Rattan, V. et al., 1994. Effect of combined supplementation of magnesium oxide and pyrodoxine in calcium-oxalate stone formers. Urol Res 22(3):161-5.

Blacklock, N. J. 1987. Sucrose and idiopathic renal stone. Nutr Health, 5(1): 9-17.

Gannon, M. C., Nuttall, F. Q. 2004. Effect of a High-Protein, Low-Carbohydrate Diet on Blood Glucose Control in People With Type 2 Diabetes. Diabetes 53(9):2375-2382.

Gannon, M. C., An increase in dietary protein improves the blood glucose response in persons with type 2 diabetes. Am J Clin Nutr 78(4):734-741.

Altorf-van der Kuil, W., et al., 2010. Dietary protein and blood pressure: a systematic review. PLoS One 5(8):e12102.

Layne, J. E., and M. E. Nelson. 1999. The effect of progressive resistance training on bone density: A Review. Medicine and Science in Sports and Exercise 31:25-30.

Zamzam K. Roughead, et al., 2003. "Controlled High Meat Diets Do No Affect Calcium Retention or Indices of Bone Status in Healthy Postmenopausal Women," The Journal of Nutrition 133, no. 4.

Terracciano, C., et al., 2013. Differential features of muscle fiber atrophy in osteoporosis and osteoarthritis. Osteoporos Int. 24(3):1095-100.

Wolfson L, Judge J, Whipple R, King M. 1995. Strength is a major factor in balance, gait, and the occurrence of falls. J Gerontol 50:64–7.

Munger, R. G., et al., 1999. Prospective study of dietary protein intake and risk of hip fracture in postmenopausal women. Amer J Clin Nutr, 69:1:147-52

Hannan, M. T. et al., 2000. "Effect of Dietary Protein on Bone Loss in Elderly Men and Women: The Framingham Osteoporosis Study," Journal of Bone and Mineral Research 15, no. 12:2504-2512.

Dawson-Hughes, B., et al., 2004. Effect of Dietary Protein Supplements on Calcium Excretion in Healthy Older Men and Women. The Journal of Clinical Endocrinology & Metabolism 89(3).

Rosenvinge Skov, A. et al., 2002. "Effect of Protein Intake on Bone Mineralization during Weight Loss: A 6-Month Trial," Obesity Research 10, no. 6:432-438.

Kerstetter, J. E., et al., 2011. Dietary protein and skeletal health: a review of recent human research. Curr Opin Lipidol. 22(1):16-20.

Hanna, M. T. et al., 2000. "Effect of Dietary Protein on Bone Loss in Elderly Men and Women, The Framingham Osteoporosis Study," Journal of Bone and Mineral Research 15, no. 12:2504-2512

Munger, R. G., et al., 1999. "Prospective Study of Dietary Protein Intake and Risk of Hip Fracture in Postmenopausal Women," The American Journal of Clinical Nutrition 69(1).

Kerstetter, J. E., et al. 2005. The impact of dietary protein on calcium absorption and kinetic measures of bone turnover in women. Journal of Clinical Endocrinology & Metabolism 90:26-31.

Heaney, R. P. Vitamin D and calcium interactions: functional outcomes. Am J Clin Nutr 88(2):541S-544S.

Bonjour, J. P., 2013. Nutritional disturbance in acid–base balance and osteoporosis: a hypothesis that disregards the essential homeostatic role of the kidney. British Journal of Nutrition 110(7):1168-1177.;

Rosenvinge Skov, A. et al., 2002. "Effect of Protein Intake on Bone Mineralization During Weight Loss: A 6-Month Trial," Obesity Research 10:432-438.

Sebastian, A. et al., 2002. "Estimation of the Net Acid Load of the Diet of Ancestral Pre-Agricultural Homo Sapiens and Their Hominid Ancestors," American Journal of Clinical Nutrition 76(6)1308-1316.

Koeppen, B. M. 2009. The kidney and acid-base regulation. Adv Physiol Educ 33(4):275-281.;

Fenton, T. R., et al., 2009. Meta-Analysis of the Effect of the Acid-Ash Hypothesis of Osteoporosis on Calcium Balance. Journal of Bone and Mineral Research 24(11):1835-1840.

Fenton, T. R., et al., 2009. Phosphate decreases urine calcium and increases calcium balance: a meta-analysis of the osteoporosis acid-ash diet hypothesis. Nutr J. 8:41.

Munger, R. G., 1999. Prospective study of dietary protein intake and risk of hip fracture in postmenopausal women. Amer J Clin Nutr 69:1:147-52

Promislow, J. H., et al., 2002. Protein consumption and bone mineral density in the elderly : the Rancho Bernardo Study. Am J Epidemiol. 155(7):636-44.

Remer, T. 2001. Influence of nutrition on acid-base balance – metabolic aspects. European Journal of Nutrition 40(5):214-220.

Kerstetter, J. E. et al., 2003. "Dietary Protein, Calcium Metabolism, and Skeletal Homeostasis Revisited," American Journal of Clinical Nutrition 78(3)584S-592S

Strohle, A., et al., 2010. Estimation of the diet-dependent net acid load in 229 worldwide historically studied hunter-gatherer societies. Am J Clin Nutr 91(2):406-412

197

Martinez-Zaguilan, R., et al., 1996. Acidic pH enhances the invasive behavior of human melanoma cells. Clin Exp Metastasis. 14(2):176-86.

Stein, J. et al. 2002. Internal Medicine. St. Louis: Mosby Year-Book.

De Santo, N. G., et al., 1997. Effect of an acute oral protein load on renal acidification in healthy humans and in patients with chronic renal failure. JASN 8(5):784-792

Remer, T., Manz, F. 1995. Potential renal acid load of foods and its influence on urine pH. J Am Diet Assoc. 95(7):791-7.;

Koeppen, B. M. 2009. The kidney and acid-base regulation. Adv Physiol Educ 33(4):275-281.

Robey, I. F., 2012. Examining the relationship between diet-induced acidosis and cancer. Nutrition & Metabolism 9:72.

Moellering, R. E., et al., 2008. Acid treatment of melanoma cells selects for invasive phenotypes. Clin Exp Metastasis 25(4):411-25.

Costill, D. et al. 1984. Acid-base balance during repeated bouts of exercise: Influence of Bicarbonate. International Journal of Sports Medicine 5:228-31.

Mistake #9

Smith, M. J. 2006. Sprint Interval Training – "It's a HIIT!" 1st edition 03/08. <http://www.sprinttraining.co.uk/Documents/Sprint%20Interval%20Training.pdf>

Leibel RL, Rosenbaum M, and Hirsch J. 1995. Changes in energy expenditure resulting from altered body weight. N Engl J Med 332: 621-628.

Sumithran, P., Prendergast, L., et al. 2011. Long-Term Persistence of Hormonal Adaptations to Weight Loss. The New England Journal of Medicine. 356(17), 1597-1604.

Wren, A. M., Seal, L. J., Cohen, M. A., et al. 2001. Ghrelin enhances appetite and increases food intake in humans. J Clin Endocrinol Metab. 86: 5992

Winder, W. W. et al. 1978. Time course sympathetic renal adaptation to endurance exercise training in man. Journal of Applied Physiology 45:370-74.

Medenhall, L. A., et al. 1994. Ten days of exercise training reduces glucose production and utilization during moderate-intensity exercise. American Journal of Physiology 266:E136-E143.

Richter, E. A. et al. 1998. Training effects of muscle glucose transport during exercise. Advances in Experiential and Medical Biology 441:107-16.

Whitworth, J. A., et al., 2005. Cardiovascular consequences of cortisol excess. Vasc Health Risk Manag. 1(4):291-9.

Kirschbaum, C., Wust, S., Faig, H.G., Hellhammer, D.H., 1992. Heritability of cortisol responses to human corticotropin-releas- ing hormone, ergometry, and psychological stress in humans. J. Clin. Endocrinol. Metab. 75:1526—1530.

Skoluda, N., Dettenborn, L., et al. 2011. Elevated Hair Cortisol Concentrations in Endurance Athletes. Psychoneuroendocrinology.

Davies, C.T., Few, J.D., 1973. Effects of exercise on adrenocortical function. J. Appl. Physiol. 35, 887—891.

Schwarz, L., Kindermann, W., 1990. Beta-endorphin, adrenocortico-tropic hormone, cortisol and catecholamines during aerobic andanaerobic exercise. Eur. J. Appl. Physiol. 61, 165—171.

Bonen, A. 1976. Effects of exercise on excretion rates of urinary free cortisol. Journal of Applied Physiology 40:155-58.

Scheele, K., Herzog, W., Ritthaler, G., Wirth, A., Weicker, H., 1979. Metabolic adaptation to prolonged exercise. Eur. J. Appl. Physiol. 41, 101—108.

Hackney, A.C., Viru, A., 1999. Twenty-four-hour cortisol response to multiple daily exercise sessions of moderate and high intensity. Clin. Physiol. 19, 178—182.

Daly, W., et al., 2004. Peak cortisol response to exhausting exercise: effect of blood sampling schedule. Med. Sport 8:17—20.

Gomez-Merino, et al., 2006. Comparison of systemic cytokine responses after a long distance triathlon and a 100-km run: relationship to metabolic and inflammatory processes. Eur. Cytokine Netw. 17, 117—124.

Kraemer, W.J., et al., 2008. Hormonal responses to a 160-km race across frozen Alaska. Br. J. Sports Med. 42:116— 120.

Davies, C. T. M., and J. D. Few. 1973. Effects of Exercise on adrenocortical function. Journal of Applied Physiology 35:887-91.

Black, P. H. 2006. The inflammatory consequences of psychologic stress: relationship to insulin resistance, obesity, atherosclerosis and diabetes mellitus, type II. Med Hypotheses. 67(4):879-91.

Peeke, P. M., Chrousos, G. P. 1995. Hypercortisolism and obesity. Ann N Y Acad Sci. 771:665-76.

Epel, E. S. et al., 2000. "Stress and Body Shape: Stress-Induced Cortisol Secretion Is Consistently Greater Among Women With Central Fat." Psychosomatic Medicine 62:623-632.

Boscolo, P., et al., 2011. Work stress and innate immune response. International Journal of Immunopathology and Pharmacology 24(1 Suppl):51S-54S.

Clark, E. M., et al., 2011. Children with low muscle strength are at an increased risk of fracture with exposure to exercise. J Musculoskelet Neuronal Interact. 11(2):196-202.

May RC, et al., 1996. Glucocorticoids and acidosis stimulate protein and amino acid catabolism in vivo. Kidney Int. 49(3):679–683.

Buchtal, F., and H. Schmalbruch. 1970. Contraction times and fiber type in intact human muscle. Acta Physiologica Scandanavica 79:435-40.

Adams, G. et al. 1993. Skeletal muscle myosin heavy chain composition and resistance training. Journal of Applied Physiology 74:911-15.

Historical Perspectives: Plasticity of mammalian muscle. Journal of Applied Physiology 90:1119-24.

Sullivan, V. et al. 1995. Myosin heavy chain composition in young and old rat skeletal muscle: Effects of endurance exercise. Journal of Applied Physiology 78:2115-20.

Laughlin, G. A., et al., 2008. Low Serum Testosterone and Mortality in Older Men. The Journal of Clinical Endocrinology & Metabolism 93(1).

Fukui, M., Nakamura, N., et al. 2010. Bone and Men's Health. Association between serum testosterone and bone mineral density in patients with diabetes. Clin Calcium. 20(2):206-11.

Tyndall, G. L., et al., 1996. Cortisol, testosterone, and insulin action during intense swimming training in humans. European Journal of Applied Physiology and Occupational Physiology 73(1-2):61-65

Derbre, F., et al., 2010. Androgen Responses to Sprint Exercise in Young Men. Int J Sports Med 31(5): 291-297.

Volek, J. S., et al., 1997. Testosterone and cortisol in relationship to dietary nutrients and resistance exercise. J Appl Physiol 82(1):49-54.

Cumming, D.C. et al. 1986. Reproductive hormone increases in response to acute exercise in men. Medicine and Science in Sports and Exercise 18:369-73.

Torjesen PA, Sandnes L. 2004. "Serum testosterone in women as measured by an automated immunoassay and a RIA". Clin. Chem. 50(3):678-9.

Southren AL, et al., 1967. "Mean plasma concentration, metabolic clearance and basal plasma production rates of testosterone in normal young men and women using a constant infusion procedure...". J. Clin. Endocrinol. Metab. 27(5):686–9

Tsai L, et al., 1991. Cortisol and androgen concentrations in female and male elite endurance athletes in relation to physical activity. Eur J Appl Physiol Occup Physiol. 63(3-4):308-11.

Raglin JS, Morgan WP, O'Connor PJ. 1991. Changes in mood states during training in female and male college swimmers. Int J Sports Med. 6:585-9.

Chatard JC, Atlaoui D, Lac G, Duclos M, Hooper S, Mackinnon L. 2002. Cortisol, DHEA, performance and training in elite swimmers. Int J Sports Med. 23(7):510-5.

Macpherson, R., Hazell, T., et al. 2011. Run Sprint Interval Training Improves Aerobic Performance but Not Maximal Cardiac Output. Medicine and Science in Sports and Exercise. 43(1), 115-121.

Booth FW. 1991. Molecular and cellular adaptation of muscle in response to exercise: perspectives of various models. Physiol Rev 71: 541-585.

Fox, E., et al. 1975. Frequency and duration of interval training programs and changes in aerobic power. Journal of Applied Physiology 38:481-84.

Dudley, G., W. Abraham, and R. Terjung. 1982. Influence of exercise intensity and duration on biochemical adaptations in skeletal muscle. Journal of Applied Physiology 53:844-50.

Davies, C. T. M., and A. Knibbs. 1971. The training stimulus: The effects of intensity, duration, and frequency of effort on maximum aerobic power output. Int. 2. Angew: 20:299-305.

Bjorntorp, P. 1997. Hormonal Control of Regional Fat Distribution. Hum Reprod 12 (Suppl 1):21-25.

Kannus, P. et al. 1992. Effect of one-legged exercise on strength, power, and endurance of the contralateral leg: A randomized controlled study using isometric and concentric isokinetic training. European Journal of Applied Physiology 64:117-24.

Bullough, R. C. 1995. Interaction of acute changes in exercise energy expenditure and energy intake on resting metabolic rate. American Journal of Clinical Nutrition 61:473-81

Mistake #10

Stein, J. et al. 2002. Internal Medicine. St. Louis: Mosby Year-Book.

Powers, S., J. Qundry, K. DeRuisseau, and K. Hamilton. 2004. Exercise and dietary antioxidants. Journal of Sports Sciences, 22:81-94.

Lawler, J., et al., 1993. Acute exercise and skeletal muscle antioxidant and metabolic enzymes. Effects of fiber type and age. American Journal of Physiology, 265: R1344-R1350.

Harman D. 1956. Aging: a theory based on free radical and radiation chemistry. J Gerontol. 11(3):298-300.

Hang Cui, Yahui Kong, Hong Zhang. 2011. "Oxidative Stress, Mitochondrial Dysfunction, and Aging" "Journal of Signal Transduction

Libby P. 2006. Inflammation and cardiovascular disease mechanisms. Am J Clin Nutr. 83:456S-60S.

Tontonoz P, et al., 1998. PPARgamma promotes monocyte/macrophage differentiation and uptake of oxidized LDL. Cell. 93(2):241-52.

Libby P. 2008. The molecular mechanisms of the thrombotic complications of atherosclerosis. J Intern Med. 263(5):517-27.

Laufs U, Fata VL, Plutzky J, Liao JK. 1998. Upregulation of Endotelial Nitric Oxide Synthase by HMG CoA Reductase Inhibitors. Circulation. 97:1129-1135.

Bamm VV, et al., 2003. Oxidation of low-density lipoprotein by hemoglobin–hemichrome. The International Journal of Biochemistry & Cell Biology. 35(3) 349-58.

Dizdaroglu M, Jaruga P. 2012. Mechanisms of free radical-induced damage to DNA. Free Radical Research. 46(4) 382-419.

Miyazaki H, Oh-ishi S, Ookawara T, et al. 2001. Strenuous endurance training in humans reduces oxidative stress following exhausting exercise. Eur J Appl Physiol. 84(1-2):1-6.

Palomero J, Jackson MJ. 2010. Redox regulation in skeletal muscle during contractile activity and aging. J Anim Sci. 88(4):1307-13.

Radak Z, Zhao Z, Koltai E, et al. 2012. Oxygen Consumption and Usage During Physical Exercise: The Balance Between Oxidative Stress and ROS-Dependent Adaptive Signaling. Antioxid Redox Signal.

Preiser, J. 2012. Oxidative Stress. JPEN J Parenter Enteral Nutr 36(2):147-154.

Sies H, Stahl W, Sevanian A. 2005. Nutritional, dietary and postprandial oxidative stress. J Nutr. 2005;135:969–972.

Halliwell B. 1991. Reactive oxygen species in living systems: source, biochemistry, and role in human disease. Am J Med. 91:14S–22S.

Vollaard NB, Shearman JP, Cooper CE. 2005. Exercise-induced oxidative stress:myths, realities and physiological relevance. Sports Med. 35:1045–1062.

Davies KJ, Quintanilha AT, Brooks GA, Packer L. 1982. Free radicals and tissue damage produced by exercise. Biochem Biophys Res Commun 107: 1198–1205.

Fisher-Wellman K, Bloomer RJ. 2009. Acute exercise and oxidative stress: a 30 year history. Dyn Med. 8:1

Radak Z, Chung HY, Koltai E, et al. 2008. Exercise, oxidative stress and hormesis. Ageing Res Rev. 7(1):34-42.

Dröge W. 2002. Free radicals in the physiological control of cell function. Physiol Rev. 82(1):47-95.

Radak Z, Chung HY, Goto S. 2005. Exercise and hormesis: oxidative stress-related adaptation for successful aging. Biogerontology. 6(1):71-5.

Morton JP, Kayani AC, McArdle A, et al. 2009. The exercise-induced stress response of skeletal muscle, with specific emphasis on humans. Sports Med. 39(8):643-62.

Nikolaidis MG, Paschalis V, Giakas G,et al. 2007. Decreased blood oxidative stress after repeated muscle-damaging exercise. Med Sci Sports Exerc. 39(7):1080-9.

Radak Z, Chung HY, Goto S. Systemic adaptation to oxidative challenge induced by regular exercise. Free Radic Biol Med. 2008 Jan 15;44(2):153-9.

Majerczak J, Rychlik B, Grzelak A, et al. 2010. Effect of 5-week moderate intensity endurance training on the oxidative stress, muscle specific uncoupling protein (UCP3) and superoxide dismutase (SOD2) contents in vastus lateralis of young, healthy men. J Physiol Pharmacol. 61(6):743-51.

Naviaux, R. K. 2012. Oxidative Shielding or Oxidative Stress? JPET 342(3):608-618

Knez WL, Jenkins DG, Coombes JS. 2007. Oxidative stress in half and full Ironman triathletes. Med Sci Sports Exerc. 39:283–288.

Goto C, et al., 2003. Effect of different intensities of exercise on endothelium-dependent vasodilation in humans: role of endothelium-dependent nitric oxide and oxidative stress. Circulation.108:530–535.

Knez WL, Coombes JS, Jenkins DG. 2006. Ultra-endurance exercise and oxidative damage: implications for cardiovascular health. Sports Med. 36:429–441.

Halliwell, B. 2006. Reactive Species and Antioxidants. Redox Biology Is a Fundamental Theme of Aerobic Life. Plant Physiology 141(2):312-322

Urso ML, Clarkson PM. 2003. Oxidative stress, exercise, and antioxidant supplementation. Toxicology. 189:41–54.

Naviaux, R. K. 2012. Oxidative Shielding or Oxidative Stress? JPET 342(3):608-618

Smith LL. 2000. Cytokine hypothesis of overtraining: A physiological adaptation to excessive stress? Med. Sci. Sports Exerc. 32: 317–31.

Rodman, P. S., McHenry, H. M. 1980. Bioenergetics and the origin of hominid biopedalism. Am J Phy Anthropol 52(1):103-6.

Schmid, P., et al., 2013. Mosaic Morphology in the Thorax of Australopithecus sediba. Science 340(6129)

Bailey, R. C., et al., 1995. The level and tempo of children's physical activities: an observational study. Med Sci Sports Exerc 27(7):1033-41.

Harman, D. 1972. "A biologic clock: the mitochondria?". Journal of the American Geriatrics Society 20 (4): 145–147.

Halliwell B. 2012. "Free radicals and antioxidants: updating a personal view. Nutrition Reviews. 70(5) 257-65.

Hultman, E. 1973. Energy metabolism in human muscle. Journal of Physiology (London) 231:56

McCully, K. et al. 1991. Biological adaptations to training: implications for resting muscle fatigue . Canadian Journal of Physiology and Pharmacology, 69: 274-78.

Edwards, R. H. T. 1983. Biological bases of fatigue in exercise performance. Biochemistry of Exercise.

Johnson, L. 1987. Biology. New York: McGraw-Hill Companies

Reid MB, Khawli FA, Moody MR. 1993. Reactive oxygen in skeletal muscle. III. Contractility of unfatigued muscle. J Appl Physiol 75: 1081–1087.

Reid MB, Shoji T, Moody MR, Entman ML. 1992. Reactive oxygen in skeletal muscle. II. Extracellular release of free radicals. J Appl Physiol 73: 1805–1809,

Powers, S. K., Jackson, M. J. 2008. Exercise-Induced Oxidative Stress: Cellular Mechanisms and Impact on Muscle Force Production. Physiol Rev 88(4):1243-1276

Kondo H, Miura M, Itokawa Y. 1993. Antioxidant enzyme systems in skeletal muscle atrophied by immobilization. Pflügers Arch 422: 404–406,

Kondo H, Miura M, Itokawa Y. Oxidative stress in skeletal muscle atrophied by immobilization. Acta Physiol Scand 142: 527–528, 1991. Medline.

Kondo H, Miura M, Kodama J, Ahmed SM, Itokawa Y. 1992. Role of iron in oxidative stress in skeletal muscle atrophied by immobilization. Pflügers Arch 421: 295–297,

Kondo H, Miura M, Nakagaki I, Sasaki S, Itokawa Y. 1992. Trace element movement and oxidative stress in skeletal muscle atrophied by immobilization. Am J Physiol Endocrinol Metab 262: E583–E590.

Kondo H, Nishino K, Itokawa Y. 1994. Hydroxyl radical generation in skeletal muscle atrophied by immobilization. FEBS Lett 349: 169–172.

Reid MB. Redox modulation of skeletal muscle contraction: what we know and what we don't. J Appl Physiol 90: 724–731, 2001.

Radak Z, Chung HY, Koltai E, et al. 2008. Exercise, oxidative stress and hormesis. Ageing Res Rev. 7(1):34-42.

Patil HR, O'keefe JH, Lavie CJ, et al. 2012. Cardiovascular damage resulting from chronic excessive endurance exercise. Mo Med. 109(4):312-21.

Droge W. 2002. Free radicals is the physiological control of cell function. Physiol Rev 82: 47–95.

Kondepudi D, Prigogine I. (1999). Modern Thermodynamics from Heat Engines to Dissipative Structures. New York: Wiley.

Supinski G. 1998. Free radical induced respiratory muscle dysfunction. Mol Cell Biochem 179: 99–110.

Supinski G, et al., 1999. Extracellular calcium modulates generation of reactive oxygen species by the contracting diaphragm. J Appl Physiol 87: 2177–2185.

Haycock JW, et al., 1996. Differential susceptibility of human skeletal muscle proteins to free radical induced oxidative damage: a histochemical, immunocytochemical and electron microscopical study in vitro. Acta Neuropathol 92: 331–340.

Di Meo S, Venditti P. 2001. Mitochondria in exercise-induced oxidative stress. Biol Signals Recept 10: 125–140.

Ji LL. 1999. Antioxidants and oxidative stress in exercise. Proc Soc Exp Biol Med 222: 283–292.

Powers, S. K., Jackson, M. J. 2008. Exercise-Induced Oxidative Stress: Cellular Mechanisms and Impact on Muscle Force Production. Physiol Rev 88(4):1243-1276

Jones, N. et al. 1977. Effect of pH on cardiorespiratory and metabolic responses to exercise. Journal of Applied Physiology 43:959-64.

Huntman, E., and J. Sjoholm. 1986. Biochemical causes of fatigue. In Human Muscle Power, ed. Champaign, IL: Human Kinetics

Kiil, F. 2002. Mechanisms of transjunctional transport of NaCl, and water in proximal tubules of mammalian kidneys. Acta Physiologica Scandanavia 175:55-70

Koeppen, B. M. 2009. The kidney and acid-base regulation. Adv Physiol Educ 33(4):275-281.

De Santo, N. G., et al., 1997. Effect of an acute oral protein load on renal acidification in healthy humans and in patients with chronic renal failure. JASN 8(5):784-792

Guyton, A., and J. E. Hall. 2000. Textbook of Medical Physiology. Philadelphia: W. B. Saunders.

Costill, D. et al. 1984. Acid-base balance during repeated bouts of exercise: Influence of Bicarbonate. International Journal of Sports Medicine 5:228-31.

McCully, K. et al. 1991. Biological adaptations to training: implications for resting muscle fatigue . Canadian Journal of Physiology and Pharmacology, 69: 274-78.

Edwards, R. H. T. 1983. Biological bases of fatigue in exercise performance. Biochemistry of Exercise.

Brooks, G. A. 1985. Anaerobic threshold: Review of the concept and directions for future research. Medicine and Science in Sports and Exercise 17:22-31.

Brooks, G. A. 1986. Lactate production under fully aerobic conditions: The lactate shuttle duing rest and exercise. Federation Proceedings, 45, 2924-2929.

Skoluda, N., Dettenborn, L., et al. 2011. Elevated Hair Cortisol Concentrations in Endurance Athletes. Psychoneuroendocrinology.

Packer, L. 1997. Oxidants, Antioxidant Nutrients, and the Athlete. Journal of Sports Science. 15(3), 353-363.

Shojaei, E., Farajoy, A., et al. 2011. Effect of Moderate Aerobic Cycling on Some Systemic Inflammatory Markers in Healthy Active Collegiate Men. International Journal of General Medicine. 24(2), 79-84.

Cakir-Atabek, H., et al., 2010. Effects of Different Resistance Training Intensity on Indices of Oxidative Stress. Journal of Strength and Conditioning Research. 24(9), 2491-2498.

Nieman, D.C. 1994. Exercise, infection, and immunity. International Journal of Sports Medicine 15:S131-S141.

Shephard, R. J., and P. N. Skek. 1995. Exercise, aging, and immune function. International Journal of Sports Medicine 16:1-6.

Walsh, N., Gleeson, M., et al. 2011. Position Statement. Part One: Immune Function and Exercise. Exercise Immunology Review. 17, 6-63.

Gleeson, Michael. 2007. Immune Function in Sport and Exercise. Journal of Applied Physiology. 103(2), 693-699.

Mackinnon LT, Hooper SL. 1996. Plasma glutamine and upper respiratory tract infection during intensified training in swimmers. Med. Sci. Sports Exerc. 28: 285–90.

Urhausen A, Gabriel H, Kindermann W. 1995. Blood hormones as markers of training stress and overtraining. Sports Med. 20: 251–76.

Lehmann M, Foster C, Dickhuth HH, Gastmann U. 1998. Autonomic imbalance hypothesis and overtraining syndrome. Med. Sci. Sports Exerc. 30: 1140–5.

Tikkanen HO, Helenius I. 1994. Asthma in runners. BMJ 309: 1087.

Cumming DC, et al. 1983. Exercise and reproductive function in women. Prog Clin Biol Res. 117: 113.

Cumming DC, et al. 1985. Defects in pulsatile release in normally menstruating runners. J Clin Endocrin Metab 60: 810.

Reid RL, van Vugt DA. 1987. Weight-related changes in reproductive function. Fertil Steril 48(6): 905.

Loucks, A. B. 2001. Physical health of the female athlete: observations, effects, and causes of reproductive disorders. Canadian Journal of Applied Physiology, 26: S176-85.

Weicker, H. et al. 1984. Changes in sexual hormones with female top athletes. International Journal of Sports Medicine, 5:200-02.

Loucks, A., and S. Horvarth. 1985. Athletic amenorrhea: A review. Medicine and Science in Sports and Exercise 17:56-72.

Dale, E., D. Gerlach, and A. Wilhute. 1979. Menstrual dysfunction in distance runners. Obestetrics and Gynecology 54:47-53.

Bullen, B. et al. 1985. Induction of menstrual disorders by strenuous exercise in untrained women. New England Journal of Medicine 312:1349-53.

De Cree, C. 1998. Sex steroid metabolism and menstrual irregularities in the exercise female: A review. Sports Medicine, 25:369-406.

Borer, K. T., 2005. Physical activity in the prevention and amelioration of osteoporosis in women: interaction of mechanical, hormonal and dietary factors. Sports Medicine 35(9):779-830.

Drinkwater, B., et al. 1984. Bone Mineral Content of amenorrheic and eumenorrheic athletes. New England Journal of Medicine 311:277-81.

Drinkwater, B. 1990. Menstrual history as a determinant of current bone density in young athletes. Journal of the American Medical Association 263:345-48.

De Souza, M.J. et al. 1994. Gonadal hormones and semen quality in male runners. International Journal of Sports Medicine, 15: 383-91.

Loucks, A. et al. 1992. The reproductive system and exercise in women. Medicine and Science in Sports and Exercise 24:S288-293.

Manna, I., Jana, K., Samanta, P. 2004. Intensive Swimming Exercise-Induced Oxidative Stress and Reproductive Dysfunction in Male Wistar Rats: Protective Role of Alpha-Tocopherol Succinate. Canadian Journal of Applied Physiology. 29(2), 172-185.

Jana, K., et al. 2008. Protective Effect of Sodium Selenite and Zinc Sulfate on Intensive Swimming-Induced Testicular Gamatogenic and Steroidogenic Disorders in Mature Male Rats. Applied Physiology, Nutrition, and Metabolism 33(5), 903-914.

Stewart, J. G., et al. 1984. Gastrointestinal blood loss and anemia in runner. Annals of Internal Medicine 100:843-45.

Haymes, E. M., and J. J. Lamanca. 1989. Iron loss in runners during exercise. Implications and recommendations. Sports Medicine 7:277-85.

Ehn, L, B. Carlwark, and S. Hoglund. 1980. Iron status in athletes involved in intense physical activity. Medicine and Science in Sports and Exercise 12:61-64.

Supinski G. 1998. Free radical induced respiratory muscle dysfunction. Mol Cell Biochem 179: 99–110.

Diaz PT, et al., 1993. Hydroxylation of salicylate by the in vitro diaphragm: evidence for hydroxyl radical production during fatigue. J Appl Physiol 75: 540–545.

Dempsey, J., and R. Fregosi. 1985. Adaptability of the pulmonary system to changing metabolic requirements. American Journal of Cardiology 55:59D-67D

Johnson, B., et al., Respiratory muscle fatigue during exercise: Implications for performance. Medicine and Science in Sports and Exercise 28:1129-37.

Dempsey, J. et al. 2003. Pulmonary limitations to exercise in health. Canadian Journal of Applied Physiology 28 (Suppl):S2-S24.

Sheppard, M. N. 2012. The fittest person in the morgue? Histopathology 60(3):381-96.

Mohlenkamp, S., et al., 2008. Running: the risk of coronary events: prevalence and prognostic relevance of coro- nary atherosclerosis in marathon runners. Eur. Heart J. 29:1903-1910.

Knez WL, Coombes JS, Jenkins DG. 2006. Ultra-endurance exercise and oxidative damage: implications for cardiovascular health. Sports Med. 36(5):429-41.

Lee IM, Hsieh CC, Paffenbarger RS., Jr 1995. Exercise intensity and longevity in men. The Harvard Alumni Health Study. JAMA. 273:1179–1184.

Quinn TJ, et al., 1990. Caloric expenditure, life status, and disease in former male athletes and non-athletes. Med Sci Sports Exerc. 22:742–750.

O'Keefe, J. H., et al. 2012. Potential Adverse Cardiovascular Effects From Excessive Endurance Exercise. Mayo Clinic Proceedings, 87(6).

O'keefe JH, Patil HR, Lavie CJ, et al. 2012. Potential adverse cardiovascular effects from excessive endurance exercise. Mayo Clin Proc. 87(6):587-95.

Sharma, S., Zaida, A. 2011. Exercise-Induced Arrhythmogenic Right Ventricular Cardiomyopathy: Fact or Fallacy. European Heart Journal.

George, K., et al., 2012. The endurance athletes heart: acute stress and chronic adaptation. Br J Sports Med. Br J Sports Med 46:i29-i36

Saltin B, Stenberg J. 1964. Circulatory response to prolonged severe exercise. J Appl Physiol 19:833–8.

La Gerche A, Connelly KA, Mooney DJ, et al. 2008. Biochemical and functional abnormalities of left and right ventricular function after ultra-endurance exercise. Heart 94:860–6.

Oxborough D, Shave R, Warburton D, et al. 2011. Dilatation and dysfunction of the right ventricle immediately after ultraendurance exercise: exploratory insights from conventional two-dimensional and speckle tracking echocardiography. Circulation: Cardiovasc Imaging 4:253–63.

Oxborough D, Whyte G, Wilson M, et al. 2010. A depression in left ventricular diastolic filling following prolonged strenuous exercise is associated with changes in left atrial mechanics. J Am Soc Echocardiogr 23:968–76.

La Gerche, A., Burns, A., et al. 2011. Exercise-Induced Right Ventricular Dysfunction and StructuralRemodeling in Endurance Athletes. European Heart Journal.

Chan-Dewar F, et al., 2010. Evidence of increased electro-mechanical delay in the left and right ventricle after prolonged exercise. Eur J Appl Physiol 108:581–7.

Chan-Dewar F, Gregson W, Whyte G, et al. 2011. Cardiac electromechanical delay is increased during recovery from 40 km cycling but is not mediated by exercise intensity. Scand J Med Sci Sports 13.

Neilan TG, Yoerger DM, Douglas PS, et al. 2006. Persistent and reversible cardiac dysfunction among amateur marathon runners. Eur Heart J 27:1079–84.

Shave R, Baggish A, George K, et al. 2010. Exercise-induced cardiac troponin elevation: evidence, mechanisms and implications. J Am Coll Cardiol 56:169–76.

Whyte GP. 2008. Clinical significance of cardiac damage and changes in function after exercise. Med Sci Sports Exerc 40:1416–23.;

Sahlen A, Gustafsson TP, Svensson JE, et al. 2009. Predisposing factors and consequences of elevated biomarker levels in long-distance runners aged >55 years. Am J of Cardiol 104:1434–40.

Mehta R, Gaze D, Mohan S, et al. 2012. Post-exercise cardiac troponin release is related to exercise training history. Int J Sports Med 33:333–7.

Middleton N, George K, Whyte G, et al. 2008. Cardiac troponin T release is stimulated by endurance exercise in healthy humans. J Am Coll Cardiol 52:1813–14.

Wilson M, O'Hanlon R, Prasad S, et al. 2009. Myocardial fibrosis in an veteran endurance athlete. BMJ Case Rep piibcr121345.

Whyte G, Sheppard M, George K, et al. 2009. Post-mortem evidence of idiopathic left ventricular hypertrophy and idiopathic interstitial myocardial fibrosis: is exercise the cause? BMJ Case Rep piibcr0820080758.

Benito B, Gay-Jordi G, Serrano-Mollar A, et al. 2011. Cardiac arrhythmogenic remodeling in a rat model of long-term intensive exercise training/clinical perspective. Circulation 123:13–22.

Breuckmann F, Möhlenkamp S, Nassenstein K, et al. 2009. Myocardial late gadolinium enhancement: prevalence, pattern, and prognostic relevance in marathon runners. Radiology 251:50–7.

Wilson MG, O'Hanlon R, Prasad S, et al. 2011. Diverse patterns of myocardial fibrosis in lifelong, veteran endurance athletes. J Appl Physiol 110:1622–6.

Mont L, Sambola A, Brugada J, et al. 2002. Long-lasting sport practice and lone atrial fibrillation. Eur Heart J 23:477–82.

Molina L, Mont L, Marrugat J, et al. 2008. Long-term endurance sport practice increases the incidence of lone atrial fibrillation in men: a follow-up study. Europace 10:618–23.

Mont L, Elosua R, Brugada J. 2009. Endurance sport practice as a risk factor for atrial fibrillation and atrial flutter. Europace 11:11–17.

Neilan TG, Yoerger DM, Douglas PS, et al. 2006. Persistent and reversible cardiac dysfunction among amateur marathon runners. Eur Heart J 27:1079–84.

Schultz, R. L., et al. 2007. Effects of Excessive Long-Term Exercise on Cardiac-Function and Myocyte Remodeling in Hypertensive Heart Failure Rats. Hyptertension 50:410-416.

O'Keefe, J. H., et al., 2012. Potential Adverse Cardiovascular Effects From Excessive Endurance Exercise. Mayo Clinic Proceedings, 87(6).

Harman D. 2009. Origin and evolution of the free radical theory of aging: a brief personal history, 1954–2009. Biogerontology. 10(6) 773-81.

Ames, B. N., et al., 1995. The causes and prevention of cancer. PNAS 92(12):5258-5265.

Diaz, M. N., et al., 1997. Antioxidants and Atherosclerotic Heart Disease. N Engl J Med 337:408-44.

Christen, Y. 2000. Oxidative stress and Alzheimer disease. Am J Clin Nutr 71(2):621s-629s.

Lang, A. E., Lozano, A. M. 1998. Parkinson's Disease. N Engl J Med 339:1044-1053

Wei, Y. H., et al., 2001. Mitochondrial theory of aging matures--roles of mtDNA mutation and oxidative stress in human aging. Zhonghua Yi Xue Za Zhi (Taipei). 64(5):259-70.

Chrousos, G.P., 2009. Stress and disorders of the stress system. Nat. Rev. Endocrinol. 5, 374—381.

McEwen, B.S., 2003. Interacting mediators of allostasis and allostatic load: towards an understanding of resilience in aging. Metabolism 52, 10—16.;

Starkie, R., M. et al., 1999. Effect of temperature on muscle metabolism during submaximal exercise in humans. Experimental Physiology 84:775-84.

Zuo, L. et al. 2000. Intra- and extracellular measurement of reactive oxygen species produced during heat stress in diaphragm muscle. American Journal of Physiology 279:C1058-66.

Marzatico, F., Pansarasa, O., et al. 1997. Blood Free Radical Antioxidant Enzymes and Lipid Peroxides Following Long-Distance and Lactacidemic Performances in Highly Trained and Aerobic and Sprint athletes. Journal of Sports Medicine and Physical Fitness. 37, 235-239.

Williams, P. T., Thompson, P. D. 2013. Walking versus running for hypertension, cholesterol, and diabetes mellitus risk reduction. Arterioscler Thromb Vasc Biol. 33(5):1085-91.

Made in the USA
San Bernardino, CA
01 December 2015